Little, Brown's Paperback Book Series
Little, Brown and Company
34 Beacon Street
Boston, Massachusetts 02106

Basic Medical Sciences

Colton	Statistics in Medicine
Hine & Pfeiffer	Behavioral Science
Kent	General Pathology: A Programmed Text
Levine	Pharmacology
Peery & Miller	Pathology
Richardson	Basic Circulatory Physiology
Selkurt	Physiology
Sidman & Sidman	Neuroanatomy: A Programmed Text
Siegel, Albers, et al.	Basic Neurochemistry
Snell	Clinical Anatomy for Medical Students
Snell	Clinical Embryology for Medical Students
Valtin	Renal Function
Watson	Basic Human Neuroanatomy

Clinical Medical Sciences

Clark & MacMahon	Preventive Medicine
Eckert	Emergency-Room Care
Grabb & Smith	Plastic Surgery
Green	Gynecology
Judge & Zuidema	Methods of Clinical Examination
Keefer & Wilkins	Medicine
MacAusland & Mayo	Orthopedics
Nardi & Zuidema	Surgery
Niswander	Obstetrics
Thompson	Primer of Clinical Radiology
Ziai	Pediatrics

Manuals and Handbooks

Arndt	Manual of Dermatologic Therapeutics
Berk et al.	Handbook of Critical Care
Children's Hospital Medical Center, Boston	Manual of Pediatric Therapeutics
Clawson & Iversen	Manual of Orthopaedic Therapeutics
Condon & Nyhus	Manual of Surgical Therapeutics
Friedman & Papper	Problem-Oriented Medical Diagnosis
Gardner & Provine	Manual of Acute Bacterial Infections
Massachusetts General Hospital	Diet Manual
Massachusetts General Hospital	Manual of Nursing Procedures
Neelon & Ellis	A Syllabus of Problem-Oriented Patient Care
Papper	Manual of Medical Care of the Surgical Patient
Shader	Manual of Psychiatric Therapeutics
Spivak & Barnes	Manual of Clinical Problems in Internal Medicine: Annotated with Key References
Wallach	Interpretation of Diagnostic Tests
Washington University Department of Medicine	Manual of Medical Therapeutics
Zimmerman	Techniques of Patient Care

TECHNIQUES OF PATIENT CARE

TECHNIQUES OF PATIENT CARE

A MANUAL OF BEDSIDE PROCEDURES
SECOND EDITION

CLARENCE E. ZIMMERMAN, M.D.
Assistant Professor of Surgery, Harvard Medical School; Associate in Surgery, Beth Israel Hospital, Boston

FOREWORD BY FRANCIS D. MOORE, M.D.
Elliott Carr Cutler Professor of Surgery, Harvard Medical School; Surgeon, Peter Bent Brigham Hospital, Boston

ILLUSTRATIONS BY TEHRIE HOLDEN

Little, Brown and Company, Boston

Copyright © 1970, 1976 by Little, Brown and Company (Inc.)
Second Edition

All rights reserved. No part of this book may be reproduced in any form or by any electronic or mechanical means, including information storage and retrieval systems, without permission in writing from the publisher, except by a reviewer who may quote brief passages in a review.

Library of Congress Catalog Card No. 75-41574

ISBN 0-316-98868-5

Printed in the United States of America

CONTENTS

Foreword by *Francis D. Moore* vii
Preface ix

1. **INTRODUCTION** 1
    1.1. Skin Preparation 2
    1.2. Infiltration Techniques 4

2. **VENOUS AND ARTERIAL TECHNIQUES** 9
    2.1. Venipuncture 9
    2.2. Arterial Punctures 16
    2.3. Intravenous Infusions 19
    2.4. Subclavian Vein Catheterization 27
    2.5. Swan-Ganz Catheter Placement 31
    2.6. Venous Cutdowns 36
    2.7. Arterial Cutdowns 46

3. **ASPIRATION TECHNIQUES** 55
    3.1. Thoracentesis 55
    3.2. Thoracostomy 63
    3.3. Pericardial Puncture 72
    3.4. Abdominal Paracentesis 74
    3.5. Culdocentesis 79
    3.6. Joint Aspiration and Synovial Biopsy 80

4. **BIOPSY TECHNIQUES** 87
    - 4.1. Bone Marrow Aspiration and Biopsy 87
    - 4.2. Vim-Silverman Needle Biopsy 93
    - 4.3. Needle Biopsy of the Liver 95
    - 4.4. Pleural Biopsy 101
    - 4.5. Collection of Cytology Specimens 104

5. **ENDOSCOPY** 111
    - 5.1. Indirect Laryngoscopy 111
    - 5.2. Bedside Bronchoscopy 113
    - 5.3. Proctosigmoidoscopy 128
    - 5.4. Fiberoptic Gastroscopy 133

6. **RESPIRATORY TECHNIQUES** 139
    - 6.1. Nasal Oxygen Catheters 139
    - 6.2. Endotracheal Suction 140
    - 6.3. Transtracheal Cough Catheter 144
    - 6.4. Emergency Tracheostomy 147

7. **NASAL PACKING** 159

8. **NASOGASTRIC INTUBATION** 165

9. **LUMBAR PUNCTURE** 177

10. **URETHRAL CATHETERIZATION** 185
    Suprapubic Intracath or Needle Drainage 195

11. **DIALYSIS TECHNIQUES** 199
    - 11.1. Peritoneal Dialysis 199
    - 11.2. Tenckoff Catheter 201
    - 11.3. Insertion of Scribner Shunt 203

12. **DRESSING CARE** 211
    - 12.1. Incision and Wound Care 211
    - 12.2. Drain Care 218
    - 12.3. Stoma Care 226

13. **TECHNIQUES OF RESUSCITATION** 235

Index *263*

FOREWORD

MODERN SURGERY has developed extremely effective tools for the hospital management of critically ill patients. Most of these methods consist in the establishment of the patient and a therapeutic modality. To achieve this interface between the outside world and the internal environment of the patient requires a whole variety of procedures which are surgical in the sense that they are performed by the hands, as skilled acts. Many of them might be thought of as minor surgery because they employ small incisions, anesthesia by the local infiltration of procaine, and only a few moments' work by the more humble members of the surgical hierarchy.

But to the patient's comfort, and to his well-being, and as a threat to the bacteriologic integrity of his internal environment, these procedures are major. If they are improperly done, they are a source of fear, insecurity, and infection. If they are properly done, then the difficulty of the principal illness or the terror of the operation immediately diminishes to manageable dimensions. Dr. Zimmerman's book is entirely devoted to the achievement of excellence in these small procedures that make major care so effective.

Using this book as a guide, the medical student, intern,

or junior resident can carry out these procedures skillfully and gently, secure in the knowledge that the directions he is following are the most effective. This confidence radiates to the patient, who in turn feels more confident when he has the freedom from discomfort and facilitation of care that these procedures all bring to him.

These are the procedures of "bedside surgery," although many of them are carried out in the operating room or in the emergency ward. This book describes a large number of these procedures. The book is very complete; and yet no two experts might agree on each detail of method shown here, and each consultant might add one or two more procedures. Those described here have emerged as successful from many years of trial and experience. Variations have been explored, and the utility of these methods established.

For me, it has been a pleasure to see the book reach this second edition because of our increasing awareness that in the skill of these minor procedures lies the secret of success for recovery after major surgery.

Francis D. Moore, M.D.

PREFACE

THE INFORMATION within the covers of this book is traditionally passed by word of mouth from generation to generation of students and house officers, and it was thus that I learned it. This method has proved adequate for the propagation of folklore, but it has several inherent weaknesses which convinced me to attempt a practical summary of bedside procedures at the conclusion of my residency in surgery, a time of peak skill in these techniques.

Now, having moved an additional five years from the "pinnacle" of bedside skills, I am more aware that bedside surgery is not immune from fashion. Techniques such as subclavian vein catheterization are in vogue and offer certain real advantages in terms of speed and effectiveness. However, before such older procedures as high cephalic venous cutdowns are abandoned, it would be well to consider that older techniques, in any given circumstances, may offer individual advantages that outweigh those of newer approaches. The physician would do well to weigh in his own mind the goals of therapy and the potential hazards of his individual approach before relegating tried-and-true techniques to premature obsolescence. This second edition of *Techniques of Patient Care* adds only those procedures that I believe offer significant new skills for the physician.

As in the first edition, coverage is limited to those procedures that can be performed at the patient's bedside; they are common, relatively simple, and important—occasionally life-saving. One's natural tendency on first attempt is to do them incorrectly, and thus to magnify their difficulty and to set the stage for further problems. When there are "tricks" that will ease technical performance, they are elaborated, but alternate solutions, contraindications, preparation, and maintenance are equally stressed because they are equally necessary for success.

Description is detailed, including a complete list of equipment required for each technique. When I was a medical student a well-meaning resident advised me to insert intravenous needles with the bevel down. The hours of frustration engendered by that piece of misinformation convinced me that such minor points need elaboration. It would be naive, however, to insist that the methods described are the only acceptable approaches. As far as possible, these techniques have been selected on the basis of effectiveness, simplicity, safety, and the lack of need for special instruments or skills. Kits at any hospital may vary the basic instruments I have listed in the text. I do not consider the contents of this book either surgically or medically oriented. With few exceptions the procedures described should be familiar ones to anyone with clinical responsibility.

Finally, I am in debt to contemporaries and residents on the Beth Israel medical, surgical and nursing staffs who assisted me in bring to this volume new techniques and procedures. I thank them collectively. Miss Tehrie Holden, the illustrator, continued to make clear technical points that are difficult to describe. The enthusiasm of Dr. Francis D. Moore during the writing of the initial edition of *Techniques of Patient Care* will always be germinal in its ultimate success.

C. E. Z.

Boston

TECHNIQUES OF PATIENT CARE

INTRODUCTION

THE TECHNIQUES described in this book include all the common procedures performed at the patient's bedside by his medical or surgical attendants. Expertness in each instance is gained only through repeated exposure, and no regrets or qualms should be felt by the beginning practitioner about early technical incompetence. This incompetence is in the nature of the learning experience, and it is modified but slightly by such physical attributes as "dexterity." Conceptual errors, however, can ruin the efforts of the most agile, or lead to a maneuver with potentially harmful consequences for the patient. The usefulness of this book lies in its ability to point out these errors.

Because the techniques described are common, they will constitute a major portion of the patient's total hospital experience. His or her cooperation will make the performance of any one of these procedures easier, yet each procedure involves varying degrees of discomfort, and its therapeutic value or diagnostic importance might not be apparent. The resolution of this dilemma lies in explanation. Above all, patients desire to become well, and if the procedure is logically related to the diagnosis and eradication of their disease, they will cooperate. This is totally the physician's responsibility, and he must never be so concerned about his abilities to perform the technique—even for the first time—that he neglects a few preliminary words of encouragement and explanation. Anything less than this might well be interpreted by the patient as unwarranted bodily assault; the doctor who arrives silently in the early morning and immediately proceeds with the passage of a nasogastric tube is asking for problems. The doctor should not gloss over possible discomfort, but he should prepare the patient for it. Pain from a "painless" procedure can cause anger and loss of confidence, but complaints are unlikely if there is less discomfort than predicted.

Bedside stands should be arranged so that the instruments within the sterile kits are in easy reach at all times, and lighting should be optimally positioned before beginning. In the middle of a thoracentesis, one has only to gaze across the room at the thoracentesis flask, out of reach, to become convinced of this fact. Time procedures, whenever possible, for maximal help, i.e., not when floor nurses are changing shifts.

1.1. SKIN PREPARATION

For the techniques requiring skin cleansing, two sterile sponges soaked in alcohol or aqueous iodine will be adequate in all cases involving needle puncture of the skin. After he has put on sterile gloves, the doctor places a sponge soaked in one of these agents over the proposed site of puncture and works outward in a spiral fashion; this process is repeated once. A dye marker will help to avoid skipping areas, and care should be taken not to touch the center of the spiral with the sponge after it has been used on the periphery. Recleansing after beginning a procedure almost invariably results in contamination; when the possibility exists that more than one needle pass will be required, as for a lumbar puncture or thoracentesis, a suitably broad area should be prepared.

When a cutdown or other linear incision is to be made, alternating swabs of aqueous iodine and alcohol may be used. To prevent iodine burns, alcohol is used for the final swab, and care is taken to prevent pooling of iodine beneath the patient; a nonirritating iodine preparation such as Betadine may be employed. Swabs are held in each hand and are worked perpendicularly away from the proposed line of incision, while the crossed hands move parallel to this line (Figure 1.1). After a single pass, the sponges are discarded

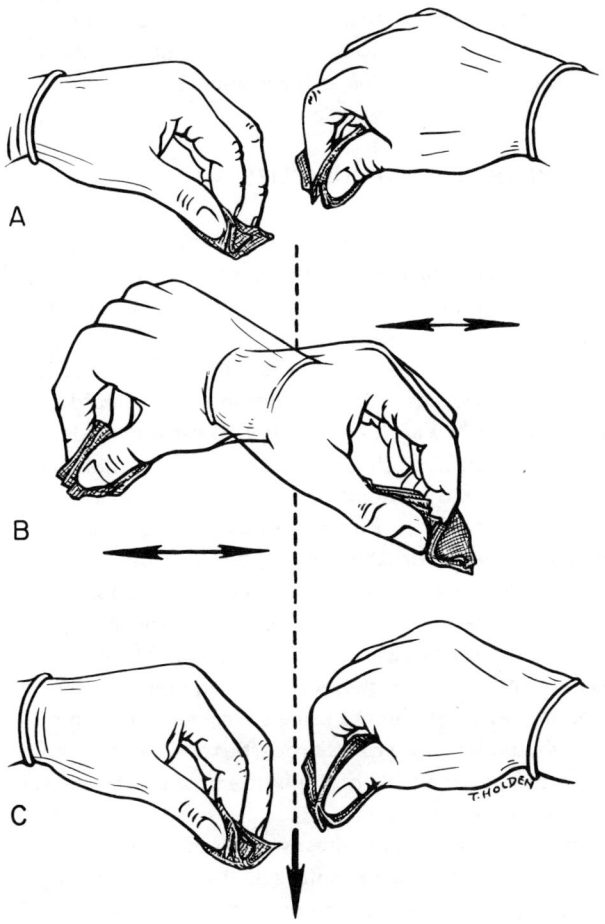

Figure 1.1.

Preparation for a linear incision. The sponges wipe at right angles away from the proposed incision, crossing slightly, while the hands move along its long axis.

3

and the alternate solution is used. The mechanical cleansing action of the sponges themselves is important, and the scrub should be performed with firm pressure against the skin. Six separate passes will adequately prepare the surface.

A true surgical field at the bedside is impossible, and the towels used to drape off the cleansed area should be placed both to avoid accidental contamination of the area and to provide a convenient surface for instruments. Because so many of the techniques to be described are done without assistance, logistic planning assumes importance.

1.2. INFILTRATION TECHNIQUES

Few of the procedures require premedication, and for some it is contraindicated. When useful, the individual chapters discuss appropriate drugs and dosages. Excessive premedication should always be avoided.

When employing local anesthetics, the smallest effective volume of the weakest effective concentration should always be used. Not only will this precaution lower the incidence of toxic reactions, but also, in the case of infiltration anesthesia, it will avoid obliteration of valuable landmarks. The use of 1% Novocain (procaine hydrochloride) or 1% Xylocaine (lidocaine) Hydrochloride will provide adequate infiltration anesthesia for all techniques in this book requiring it. The addition of epinephrine prolongs the effectiveness of these agents through the mechanism of vasoconstriction, but this effect is not required for any procedure described. Before using a local anesthetic the doctor should be aware of its properties and toxicity, and he should check the label of the bottle or vial before drawing the agent into his syringe.

A rare individual will manifest severe sensitivity to a particular anesthetic agent. Before he uses any such drug, the doctor should question the patient specifically about previous untoward reactions. These unfavorable responses can be severe, and can include central nervous system stimulation or depression, peripheral vascular collapse, and allergic reactions. Resuscitation equipment should be available (see Chapter 13, Techniques of Resuscitation), in case respiratory assistance and supplemental oxygen are required. Intravenous amobarbital or thiopental in small amounts may be used to control convulsions; intravenous vasopressors will be indicated for peripheral vascular collapse; and epinephrine, with or without an antihistamine such as Benadryl (diphenhydramine hydrochloride), is effective against allergic manifestations. Common agents and dosages are listed. These are suggested and safe ranges for average adults. Smaller amounts are indicated for children, the elderly, and the severely debilitated.

INFILTRATION ANESTHETICS

1. Xylocaine (lidocaine) Hydrochloride, in a 0.5 to 2% solution. Safe dosage range is 40 to 50 ml of the 1% and 20 to 25 ml of the 2% solution.
2. Novocain (procaine hydrochloride) in a 0.5 to 2% solution. Although potency is considered less than lidocaine, dosage range is the same.
3. Carbocaine (mepivacaine hydrochloride), 1 and 2% solutions available. Similar dosage range to lidocaine.
4. Cyclaine (hexylcaine hydrochloride), 1% solution. Safe limit is 40 ml.

TOPICAL ANESTHETICS

1. Xylocaine (lidocaine) Hydrochloride, as a 4% solution. Up to 200 mg (5 ml), recommended maximum dose.
2. Cocaine hydrochloride, usually as a 2 to 10% solution. Maximum recommended dosage to 300 mg.
3. Pontocaine Hydrochloride (tetracaine hydrochloride), in a 0.1 to 2% solution. Dosage not to exceed 40-50 mg.
4. Dyclone (dyclonine hydrochloride), in a 0.5 to 1% solution. Up to 70-80 mg is recommended maximum dosage.
5. Cyclaine Hydrochloride (hexylcaine hydrochloride), 2.5 to 5% solution. Up to 100 mg is recommended maximum dosage.

The most common error in anesthetizing the skin for puncture or incision is to deposit the bulk of the agent in the subcutaneous tissue. The vast majority of pain sensors lie within the dermis, and the initial anesthetic wheal must be intradermal to affect them. An intradermal injection causes a characteristic white distension of the skin, and a prominence of the hair follicles. It should be performed slowly; rapid distension of the skin will cause pain before the anesthetic has time to work. For this, a 25-gauge needle is desirable; of adequate bore, it is less painful than larger needles. Deeper infiltration can then be obtained using a longer 22-gauge or 20-gauge needle.

For a linear incision, the long needle is bent at the hub about 30 degrees. This will enable the operator to hold the syringe comfortably while advancing the needle *intradermally,* parallel with the skin surface. The needle is introduced at the site of the original wheal and pushed forward, while infiltrating along the projected line of incision. Progress will be easier if the skin is held taut with the free hand. Should the needle be too short, it may be reintroduced through previously anesthetized portions of the incisional ridge. At the conclusion, the anesthetic agent may then be deposited subcutaneously beneath this line.

For deeper punctures, effective anesthesia requires infiltration not only along the proposed needle tract, but also of a core of tissue about this tract approximately 1 cm in diameter. Patient movement and human error make it extremely difficult to duplicate the original needle path by

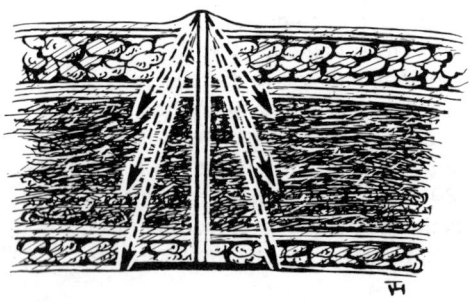

Figure 1.2.

Proper method of anesthesia infiltration for a deep needle passage. Note that a core of tissue, rather than a single track, is infiltrated.

a later one. The technique for obtaining this anesthesia is illustrated in Figure 1.2. To avoid inadvertent intravascular injections of anesthetic agents on deep passes of the needle, aspirate for blood before each injection. Periosteum, peritoneum, and pleura are pain-sensitive membranes; they must be adequately anesthetized.

2.

VENOUS AND ARTERIAL TECHNIQUES

2.1. VENIPUNCTURE

Venipuncture is likely to be one of the first tasks assigned to the medical student or intern. It can be an extremely simple or a frustratingly difficult technique, and this axiom holds true for the experienced as well as for the inexperienced practitioner. The accessibility of veins varies tremendously from patient to patient, and the proper approach to, and "feel" of, a useful vessel requires repeated practice. The beginner should feel no guilt upon missing the first few venipunctures. Unfortunately, the technique involves some pain, and many individuals have a deep-rooted fear of the hypodermic needle. Repeated attempts can lead to anxiety and anger on the part of the patient, but they must not cause hesitation if the sample is needed. Above all, the physician should not allow himself to become anxious. His chances of success will be much reduced, and he would do better to return at a later time or request more experienced help.

Ninety-five percent of venipunctures are performed on one of the several veins crossing the antecubital space, and for sound reasons. The vessels here are large and thick-walled, so that they will not collapse when blood is withdrawn, and they are relatively fixed in place. Before one looks elsewhere, this area should be inspected on both arms. Other veins used less frequently are those on the dorsum of the hand and volar surface of the wrist, the cephalic vein on the radial aspect of the wrist, the external and internal jugular veins, and the femoral vein. The last is used most often when emergency samples are required in the treatment of shock, and the technique is the same as that described for femoral artery puncture (p. 18), except that the needle is directed to the medial side of the femoral pulse. If the patient has experienced repeated venipunctures, he may well be able to direct the doctor to the vein used most successfully.

MATERIAL

Twenty-gauge needle (disposable if available). These needles are always sharp, and the danger of cross-contamination is eliminated. Avoid long bevels which might pierce the posterior wall of the vein. Also, suitably large sterile syringe, tourniquet, antiseptic-soaked sponge, dry sponge, and selected tubes or bottles for samples.

Comment. Many hospitals have now adopted for standard collections a Vacutainer system that transfers blood directly from the needle to evacuated tubes. This system uses a special double-ended needle that screws into a plastic adapter (Figure 2.1). The longer end is used for the venipuncture, and a sealed, evacuated tube, which had previously been lightly seated on the short end of the needle, is then pushed down so that the short tip punctures the rubber cap of the tube and blood is sucked into it. While generally of great usefulness, particularly when multiple samples are required, the Vacutainer system cannot be used for a few specialized studies for which red cell integrity is crucial, or during which exposure to air is not permissible, as in blood gas determinations. The laboratory supervisor can advise the physician when the Vacutainer samples are inadequate. Remember that it is impossible to use the Vacutainer system effectively in any of the secondary locations except the femoral vein. The veins are soft or small, and will collapse with the suction, shutting off flow to the needle. When

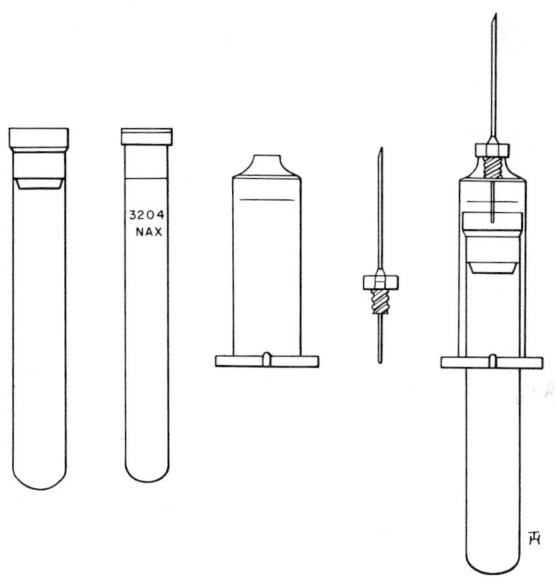

Figure 2.1.
Vacutainer system, illustrating component parts and assembled unit.

these sites are selected, a syringe and needle are employed, and suction must be slow and gentle.

TECHNIQUE
The patient is semirecumbent or supine. It is difficult to predict the psychologic and nervous reaction of an individual to venipuncture, and therefore the procedure should be briefly explained, and the patient instructed to look away during its accomplishment. If the patient is a child or infant, a nurse must be in attendance to calm or to control him.

A tourniquet is placed tightly about the upper arm as illustrated in Figure 2.2. This allows it to be pulled free with one hand without catching hairs. After about 15 seconds, the doctor should inspect the antecubital space and palpate for veins, using the balls of the second and third fingers of the free hand. The skin over the vessels is gently pressed inward, and the vein is felt as a soft but slightly elastic cord—the precise description is difficult, but mastery of the

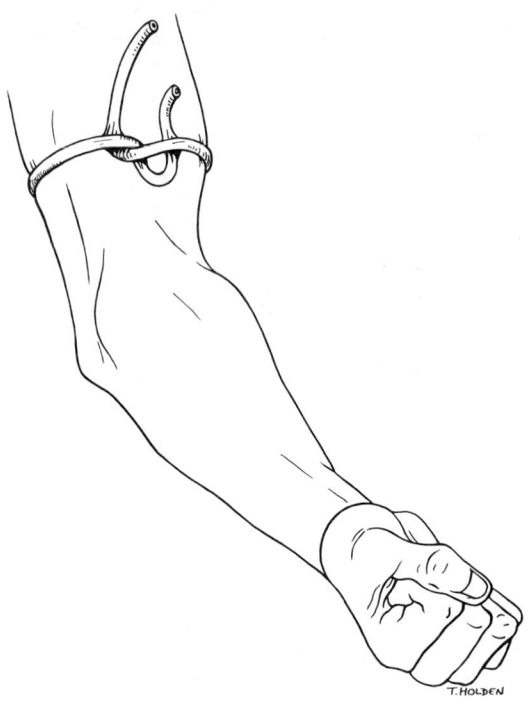

Figure 2.2.

Proper application of venous tourniquet. Repeated clenching of the fist will make veins more prominent. The medial end of the tubing in this illustration is pulled to release the tourniquet.

procedure comes with experience. The entire area is examined carefully, and if no veins are felt, it is reexamined after the tourniquet has remained in place for an additional minute, while the patient repeatedly opens and closes his hand. When a vessel is located, a careful mental picture is formed of its estimated depth and direction, and the area over it is swabbed clean. The skin over the vein is now punctured, with the needle bevel up, directly over the vessel and guided in the direction of its long axis. Piercing the skin is done rapidly, for it is painful, but then the needle is advanced slowly downward toward the vein until blood can be freely aspirated into the syringe, or the tip of the Vacutainer needle is felt to be within the lumen. Entry often may be felt as a slight but definite "give." The blood sample is aspirated slowly.

Note. If multiple tubes are used with the Vacutainer needle, it is possible to avoid leaking blood during tube changes by compressing the vein down onto the needle tip with the free hand while switching.

Before withdrawing the needle, remove the tourniquet and apply pressure over the venotomy site with a dry sponge. Maintain this pressure during withdrawal, and have the patient continue to apply it for an additional minute. Do not have him hold the sponge by folding his arm at the elbow, for this will often partially obstruct the vein above the site of entry, and will thus favor the formation of a hematoma.

If secondary sites on the wrist or dorsum of the hand are chosen, the veins may be made more prominent by snapping them sharply with the finger, or by applying hot compresses to the hand, although the latter is usually impractical. Because the loose areolar tissue surrounding the dorsal veins allows these veins to roll away from the needle point, they should be first held securely in place with the thumb of the free hand (see Figure 2.5).

External Jugular Vein Puncture

This technique is particularly useful in infants or small children when other veins are likely to be unsuitable. The child is positioned crossways on the bed or treatment table, his head hanging freely over the edge. A nurse grasps both wrists in front of him with one hand, and with the other turns the head (Figure 2.3). In this position, venous pressure in the head and neck is accentuated, and the external jugular vein usually becomes visible with respirations. Pressure in the vein and distension may be increased further by a Valsalva maneuver or breath holding, and in the infant this is accomplished by having the nurse flick the heels until the baby cries.

Stand opposite the nurse at the infant's head and direct the needle caudally (in the direction of flow), into this

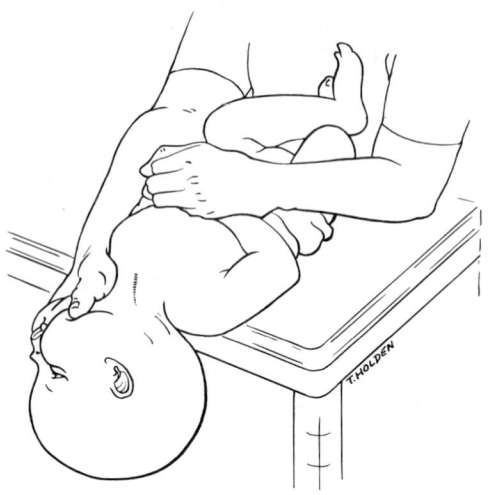

Figure 2.3.

External or internal jugular vein puncture. Infant's head is allowed to hang freely, then is turned by the assistant. If restraint is inadequate, infant should be wrapped in a sheet.

superficial vessel, piercing the skin at the level of the junction of the middle and upper thirds of the vein. Holding the syringe will be much easier if the needle (20 or 22 gauge) is first bent 45 degrees at the hub. Some prefer to use a Butterfly needle for this, and it adapts itself very nicely to the job. Even in the head-down position and with a clean venipuncture, flow will be slow and pulsate with respirations. Be gentle with aspiration, and phase it to correspond with this intermittent filling of the vein.

Internal Jugular Vein Puncture

The indications are the same as for external jugular puncture when the latter is not feasible. The infant and the physician are in the identical positions as for external vein puncture. The mastoid process and sternal notch are palpated, and an imaginary line projected between them. The needle is directed along this line with the skin penetrated at a point about 1 inch below the mastoid process, along the lateral border of the sternocleidomastoid muscle. This edge will stand out distinctly when the head is turned. Direct the needle (20 or 22 gauge, bent 45 degrees at the hub—a Butterfly needle is *not* applicable), beneath the muscle toward the sternum until the tip is palpable just above the notch. If no blood is aspirated, withdraw slowly, applying gentle suction to the syringe, and stopping at the point where blood is freely returned. Because of the proximity of other carotid sheath structures, it is essential that the infant be securely held, if necessary bound in a sheet, so that the assistant can use both hands to hold the head.

Blood Cultures

These cultures are obtained via a standard antecubital venipuncture, but special care is taken to avoid extraneous bacterial contamination of the blood during or after its withdrawal. The system described is simple, effective, and applicable in most clinical situations. An alcohol lamp is lit at the bedside, the tourniquet applied, and the vein located in the usual manner. Following this, however, *the skin is not touched with the fingers until the sample is secured,* the needle being guided from memory only. The skin over the vessel is disinfected with two swabs of aqueous iodine, followed by two of alcohol. Sterile gloves may be worn, but they are less crucial than a careful technique.

A disposable 20-gauge needle is now attached to a sterile syringe, care being taken not to touch either the needle shaft or the adapter hub of the syringe. The venipuncture is performed, 10 to 15 ml of blood obtained, and the needle withdrawn. A dry gauze is not applied to the puncture site until the needle is completely free of the skin, to avoid contamination of its tip. The needle and syringe are carefully disconnected without touching the adapter of the latter.

Whether the culture media are held in screw-cap bottles or cotton-plugged tubes, the tops of the containers are flamed in the lamp, after removing the caps or plugs, but before transferring 5 ml of blood to each container, and then are reflamed before securing them.

2.2. ARTERIAL PUNCTURES

Arterial puncture, for the obtaining of samples used in monitoring arterial blood gases, is performed on the brachial, radial, and femoral arteries. Each site has its advantages and shortcomings, and facility at all sites will be useful. When a patient is likely to require frequent samplings over a period of days, the incidence of the two major complications of this technique, thrombosis and hematoma formation, is increased, and a radial artery cutdown (Section 2.7) is a safer alternative.

MATERIAL
Disposable 20-gauge needle and 10-ml or 20-ml glass syringe (heparin coated), plastic bag or basin containing ice (large enough to hold the syringe), cork or rubber stopper, antiseptic-soaked sponges, and dry sponges.
Comment. Plastic, disposable syringes with rubber seals and considerable friction between barrel and plunger are not ideal, although they are feasible. To coat the barrel with heparin, aspirate 1 ml of heparin directly from its container (1000 USP units per milliliter), then pull back the plunger while twirling the barrel to cover the inner surface of the syringe evenly with a thin layer of the fluid. Expel all but a drop or two of heparin, allowing no air to reenter the syringe.

TECHNIQUE
Brachial Artery Puncture
The vessel is selected in the area where it crosses anterior to the medial epicondyle, prior to its bifurcation into the ulnar and radial divisions (Figure 2.4). The median nerve has crossed from the lateral to the medial side of the vessel, the brachial vein and median antebrachial cutaneous nerve are separated from it by the deep fascia, and the lacertus fibrosus intervenes between it and the venae cubiti. The relationships of the artery should be reviewed before approaching it, for although injury to these neighboring structures is unusual, their proximity is a potential hazard.

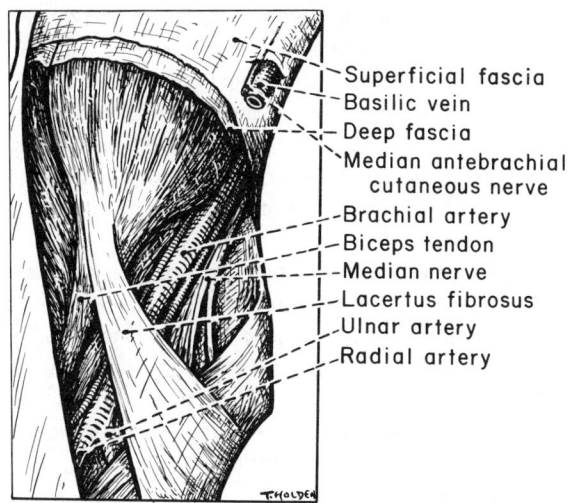

Figure 2.4.

Anatomic dissection of brachial artery, illustrating relationships of adjacent structures.

The patient is reclining, with the selected arm resting abducted, and slightly hyperextended at the elbow by a small folded towel placed behind it. A nurse should be at the patient's side to maintain pressure on the vessel after the puncture.

Feel for the pulse at the elbow. In muscular or obese individuals, the brachial pulse may not be palpable, and a puncture should not be attempted unless the pulse is well felt. Once the pulse has been located, the skin is disinfected and penetrated with the needle bevel up, and at right angles to the vessel. Hold the syringe like a large pencil; when it is thus grasped, the pulse may often be felt, transmitted to the needle, when its tip touches the vessel wall.

Advance slowly toward the pulse until bright blood pushes into the syringe. Blood under arterial pressure will push back the plunger of the syringe without aspiration; this is an excellent indication that the needle is not in a vein. Once certain of the location, withdraw 5 ml of blood and then rapidly remove the needle while compressing the artery firmly with a dry sponge, taking care not to suck air into the syringe. Occlusive pressure must be maintained a full 5 minutes *by the clock*. One of the advantages of this site is that the medial epicondyle forms a good backstop against which to compress the artery. Skewer the cork or stopper with the needle tip to prevent air aspiration, and cover the syringe with ice.

Loss of distal pulses and a cold painful hand are reported complications of this procedure, but they are almost always temporary and are thought to be secondary to arterial spasm. There is a rich collateral flow about the elbow, and should the brachial artery be thrown into spasm, these vessels theoretically could take up the load. The brachial artery should not be used repeatedly. A firm pressure dressing may be applied if oozing recurs after two 5-minute periods of compression.

Femoral Artery Puncture
The patient is recumbent. Locate the pulse just distal to the inguinal ligament. When the patient is obese, with a large panniculus, a nurse should elevate the panniculus and hold open the inguinal crease. The femoral nerve is lateral and the femoral vein medial to the pulse, and a good method of isolating the artery, after disinfecting the skin, is to place the index and middle fingers of the free hand over the nerve and vein, on either side of the pulse, and stretch the skin taut. The syringe again is held like a pencil, the needle pierces the skin between these two fingers, and advances straight for the pulse at right angles to the vessel wall. While a transmitted beat may be felt as the needle touches the artery, it is more common not to feel anything and actually not to see arterial blood pushing into the syringe until the full length of the needle has been advanced and is being withdrawn. Therefore, withdrawal should be slow, with constant rotation of the syringe as it moves. An initially unsuccessful pass may be repeated after withdrawing the needle tip to a superficial location. Stay on the lateral side of the pulse to avoid the vein and the contamination of the syringe and needle with venous blood.

Once the sample is drawn, the needle is corked and the syringe iced while an assistant maintains 5 minutes of firm pressure over the artery with a dry sponge. Even when no hematoma appears to be developing, the patient should be checked within a half hour for any subsequent bleeding, particularly if he has a clotting disorder or is on anticoagulants. Although the femoral artery may be used repeatedly with greater safety than the brachial artery, the necessity for repetition is one valid indication for an indwelling line at the wrist. Femoral artery puncture in any leg with major arterial occlusions or advanced atherosclerosis should be avoided whenever possible.

Radial Artery Puncture
Secure the wrist in the hyperextended position over a rolled towel and introduce the needle, bevel up, directly over the radial pulse, parallel with the vessel at the level of the radial styloid, and at an angle of 45 degrees with the skin. Advance the needle slowly until blood spurts into the syringe.

Five minutes of firm digital pressure and a pressure dressing are applied at the conclusion of the procedure. While the presence of the palmar vascular arches make this location perhaps the safest of the three locations described, the artery is small and easily injured, and therefore should not be used repeatedly.

Femoral artery puncture, accomplished with a 22- or 23-gauge needle and with complete immobilization of the leg by the physician, can be performed in infants. This should be done, however, only by those familiar with handling infants and familiar with the technique in adults.

Note: Blood is a living fluid. After blood remains at room temperature for over 15 minutes, the blood gas determinations are severely altered. Unless the laboratory is a few steps away, all samples should be ice cooled immediately.

2.3. INTRAVENOUS INFUSIONS

Before approaching the mechanics of this common procedure, review briefly the variables which will determine whether or not the final arrangement of tube and needle is adequate to meet the particular problem. When such considerations become automatic, subsequent revisions are rarely required.

Drugs

What drugs are to be administered? Powerful vasoactive agents such as norepinephrine, hypertonic solutions, and locally toxic drugs must not be infused through a peripheral vein, for fear of extensive necrosis should the infusion infiltrate into surrounding tissues. These solutions should be given via either a central venous catheter or a carefully monitored short catheter of the Rochester type in the antecubital vein, although the former route is safer and thus preferred.

Needles

What is the proper size and type of needle? In febrile illnesses leading to dehydration, such as pneumonia and pyelonephritis, and in diseases in which vomiting is common, such as cholecystitis, small needles of 20- or 21-gauge bore in peripheral veins are perfectly adequate, are less likely to cause phlebitis, and are often easier to position than catheters or needles of larger bore. Prepackaged disposable needles are available in all sizes; they are always sharp, and they are free from the potential hazard of transmitting infectious disease. There are three groups of patients in whom veins are notoriously difficult to cannulate: the infant (veins are small), the elderly (veins are tortuous and fragile), and the obese (superficial veins are scarce and small). With these patients, the winged Butterfly needle, available in 19- or 21-gauge bores, is preferable. Originally designed for pediatric use, this needle is the easiest to guide accurately into small vessels, and once in place it may be securely taped down.

When hemorrhage is active, *or threatened,* however, it is much wiser to choose a large-bore needle, a needle-catheter set, or a venous cutdown rather than face an early morning decision of whether or not to try to force blood through an inadequate needle. An 18-gauge bore or larger is required for rapid transfusion, but such needles may often quite easily be positioned in a peripheral vein. When the infusion is to continue for over 24 hours, and transfusion is likely, the readily available Rochester-type catheter units are highly effective and uniformly preferable to the older style Bard Intracath. This is because the needle lies within the lumen of the catheter and is completely removed following venipuncture, thereby obviating the possibility of shearing off the catheter with the needle point—a rarely reported but potentially disastrous hazard with the older unit. In addition, the catheter can be larger for any given needle size (once again, because the catheter passes around the needle rather than through it).

Veins

What are the most suitable veins for use? Although often prominent and easily cannulated, the discomfort and instability of intravenous needles in the foot render pedal veins impractical. The greater saphenous vein at the ankle can be entered percutaneously, but the restrictions to movement that this forces upon the patient, plus the rapid appearance of phlebitis, also makes this area of limited usefulness. The antecubital veins are large, accessible, and often chosen first, but there are four disadvantages to their use for continuous infusion. (1) These veins are the most valuable for drawing blood samples and will be useless for this purpose as long as the infusion is running, or if it should infiltrate. (2) The antecubital veins bridge the elbow joint, and this must be held in extension with a long board to prevent dislodgment of the needle. This position quickly will become uncomfortable. (3) Because of the depth and position of these vessels, the cannula must enter them at a considerable angle to their long axis, a position not conducive to prolonged stability. (4) This area cannot be used for monitoring the blood pressure while the infusion set is in place.

The preferred veins are those on the dorsal surface of the hand and forearm, and the volar surface of the forearm proximal to the carpal ligament (do not use the small veins directly over the volar carpal ligament, for infiltration here can and has caused median nerve injury). These veins should always be inspected first before the physician turns elsewhere.

In the infant, it may be necessary to utilize the scalp veins and the scalp vein or Butterfly needle. The baby should first be restrained with a sheet wrapping or by an assistant, and then the scalp may be shaved and scrupulously cleansed. Always shave the entire head; there is something peculiarly grotesque to parents about the sight of a half-shaved scalp. Even in the newborn, however, the dorsal veins on the hand may be surprisingly large, and a careful examination may make cannulation of the scalp veins unnecessary. Scalp veins drain deeply into the cerebral system, and an infusion must be stopped promptly at the first sign of local inflammation.

The subclavian vein may be cannulated blindly with a high degree of success, and although this vein is used primarily for monitoring central venous pressure, it can also be used for infusions. However, this rather delicate technique has resulted in pneumothorax, and it should not be attempted by the inexperienced. The patient is placed in the Trendelenburg position to make the vein distend, his head is turned to the side opposite to the vein, and the skin is pierced with a long, 11-cm Rochester-type needle on a syringe at a point one finger-breadth below the clavicle at its midpoint. The needle is then directed upward beneath the clavicle, angling for the hollow between the sternal and clavicular heads of the sternocleidomastoid muscle. When blood is returned, the needle is advanced another centimeter, then removed if flow is satisfactory. The catheter is pushed forward in the usual manner and secured. Because accidental uncoupling of the intravenous tubing and catheter hub has resulted in cases of fatal air embolism, all the junctions from the catheter hub to the intravenous bottle should be firmly taped together.

MATERIAL

Intravenous fluid bottle and parenteral administration tubing (connected and hanging from a support); 1-inch adhesive tape (in the absence of tape allergy, standard tape is preferable to the mechanically weaker nonallergenic type), pretorn and placed in strips where the strips can be easily reached; needle; 5-ml syringe partially filled with saline solution; tourniquet; lightweight padded board (about 10 inches long for the hand, 16 inches long for antecubital veins); sponge with antiseptic solution.

TECHNIQUE

Explain the procedure to the patient. *As standard procedure,* attach the saline solution-filled syringe, rather than the intravenous tubing, to the needle or needle-catheter combination. Do not jam them together too tightly; they must be disconnected later when the cannula is in the vein.

Apply the tourniquet tightly about the upper arm and have the patient dangle his arm over the side of the bed for 3 minutes, then inspect his hand and forearm for suitable vessels. Many methods, such as wrapping the extremity in a hot towel, have been described to bring surface veins into more prominence, but vessels still insignificantly small after simple proximal obstruction are generally not worth pursuing. In the hand and forearm it is possible, although difficult, to enter veins which are palpable but not visible, and those that can be seen should be approached first. A vein may be made to "stand up" more prominently by flicking it sharply with a finger, thus paralyzing its intrinsic vascular tone. This maneuver should be done immediately prior to venipuncture, for the effect is short-lived, and it may be repeated after the application of the skin cleanser, which usually causes surface cooling and vasoconstriction.

The veins on the dorsum of the hand lie immediately beneath the skin, surrounded only by loose areolar tissue that offers no resistance to free motion. It is therefore common for them to roll away easily from the advancing needle tip. To avoid this annoyance, particularly common in the elderly, in whom veins are also fragile, grasp the patient's hand with the free hand, as illustrated in Figure 2.5, and, placing the thumb over the distal end of the selected vessel, roll the loose skin downward toward the knuckles. This simple maneuver, applicable to infusions started in every location, anchors one end of the vein to prevent excessive rolling and also stabilizes the patient's hand.

When using a Butterfly needle, grasp the wings between thumb and index finger; if the Rochester catheter or needle is connected directly to the syringe, cradle the syringe in the curve of the fingers. Pass the needle, bevel up, through the skin directly over the selected vein and parallel with its long axis. Some physicians advocate introducing the needle

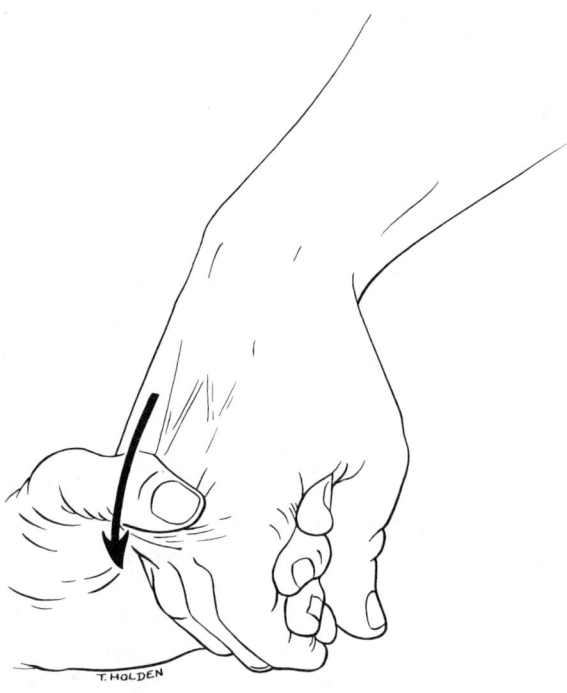

Figure 2.5.

Stabilization of the veins on the dorsum of the hand. Grasping the hand in this manner also secures the hand itself.

at a distance from the vein and then advancing it into the lumen, but the inevitable angle the cannula will thus make with the vein's long axis will tend to kink the vessel on the tip and produce early infiltration.

Advance the needle slowly on a gradually deepening course, maintaining stabilizing counteraction with the free thumb, until the tip is felt to be within the lumen (there often is a palpable "give"), then gently aspirate with the syringe if blood does not come into it spontaneously. If blood does not return on aspiration, the tip is not within the vein lumen; one should continue to advance it until blood is freely aspirated. At this point gently inject a small amount from the syringe. If the needle is properly placed, the subcutaneous tissue will not balloon up; if it does, a site further up the vein should be selected, as the presence of aspirated blood indicates vessel wall damage. The needle may be gently advanced within the lumen for added stability, although this maneuver is not essential and should not be attempted if the course of the vein is not clearly visible. When a Rochester-type catheter is being used, the cannula should be pushed forward about two centimeters after the needle is removed. Try to select a site on the dorsum of the hand that will allow the hub of the needle or the wings of the Butterfly needle to rest proximal to the knuckles, where it may be more firmly secured.

Remove the tourniquet. To secure the needle, two 2-inch lengths of adhesive strips across the exposed shaft and hub will hold it initially. Gently disengage the syringe, attach and open the I.V. tubing, and ask the patient to slowly grasp the handboard. Three strips of tape, across the hand, wrist, and forearm, respectively, will secure the board. Do not tape down the fingers unless the patient is agitated; he can move them without disturbing the needle. If the hub lies upon the knuckles, however, it will be necessary to tape the fingers in an extended position. Occasionally the fluid will run more smoothly if the hub of the needle is elevated upon a small pledget of folded tape or gauze, thereby depressing the tip into the lumen. Make a loop of the intravenous tubing and tape it to one of the securing strips on either the wrist or forearm. Thus if the patient should jerk the tubing, the tug will be stopped here rather than conducted to the needle.

The tape eventually must be removed, and the hairy areas of the wrist and forearm should be protected against this painful procedure. Gauze may be placed beneath the strips, but this precaution tends to allow too much motion. A reversed strip of tape (sticky side up), pretorn with the other pieces and lying beneath each circumferential band, is preferable. Figure 2.6 illustrates a well-secured intravenous line, with three-point fixation of the wrist, and with the thumb free.

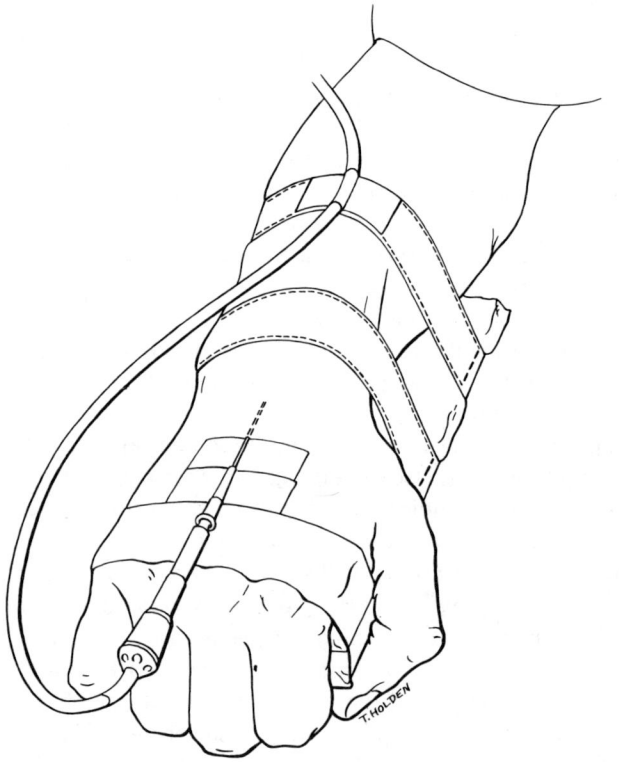

Figure 2.6.

Properly secured handboard. Note freedom of fingers and reversed tape beneath proximal two encircling strips.

If the line is in a distal vein and becomes plugged, the obstruction may often be cleared simply by balling up the intravenous tubing and giving the mass a sharp squeeze. Should this prove insufficient, disconnect the tubing and flush the needle with a syringe, preferably a tuberculin or similar small type, because the thrust delivered by it will far exceed that of a larger one.

Local pain during infusion should initially cause suspicion of infiltration. However, properly running infusions of such diverse fluids as plasma and saline solution can cause severe local discomfort in certain patients, reactions that are highly idiosyncratic. Simply slowing the drip rate often helps, and warm compresses may yield some relief in more severe cases. Potassium is a well-recognized intimal irritant, and in concentrations above 20 milliequivalents per liter it will regularly cause local pain. Such concentrations are generally avoidable.

Heparin, at 10 mg per liter of intravenous solution, may delay the onset of phlebitis, but the cannula itself may be irritating, and *each day it is in place will increase the likelihood of this complication. Remove the line at the first sign of phlebitis.*

2.4. SUBCLAVIAN VEIN CATHETERIZATION

The introduction of a polyethylene catheter into the infraclavicular portion of the subclavian vein, for central pressure monitoring or intravenous hyperalimentation, is a useful and reasonably safe procedure when performed with care and knowledge of local anatomy. The described technique is a relatively simple but accurate method for the placement of subclavian lines.

MATERIAL
Fourteen-gauge Intracath, antiseptic solution, local anesthetic and syringe, sterile sponges.

TECHNIQUE
Because in the technique described the Intracath is not opened at any point to trim catheter length or to aspirate

blood, the use of caps, gowns, and gloves is superfluous. The vein is to be punctured as it passes behind the clavicle (Figure 2.7). To distend the vein, the patient is placed in as steep a Trendelenburg's position as he can tolerate, with the face averted and with a towel roll placed between the shoulder blades (Figure 2.7). This allows the needle to be advanced in a direction away from the cupula of the lung. An area below the anterior bow of the clavicle is prepared widely and thoroughly. If desired, the puncture site is first infiltrated with local anesthetic. The Intracath needle puncture is performed at the anterior bow of the clavicle, using

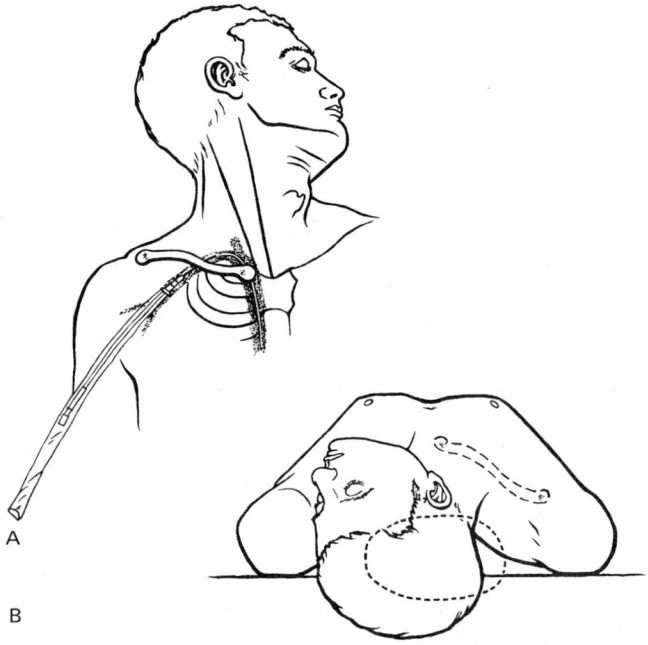

Figure 2.7.

Subclavian vein catheterization. (**A**) Intracath passage indicating relationship of subclavian vein to clavicle. The skin puncture site is at the anterior bow of the clavicle. Note also the relationship of the vein to the sternal notch. (**B**) Patient position for subclavian vein catheterization. The head is averted and a towel roll is placed between the shoulder blades to elevate the clavicle above the shoulder line. To distend the vein, the patient is also placed in as steep a Trendelenburg's position as is feasible.

the sternal notch and anterior scalene muscle as landmarks. The needle is advanced in the plane of the anterior ribs on a direct line toward the sternal notch. Advancement in the plane of the ribs avoids pulmonary complications, but if the clavicle is encountered, the needle is "walked" beneath (i.e., behind) it. After the needle has been advanced its full length, the catheter is moved forward approximately a distance of 20 cm and the needle is withdrawn. If resistance is met on catheter advancement, it is brought back to its original position with the needle still in place. The entire unit is now withdrawn several centimeters and advanced in a slightly deeper plane, and the catheter moved forward again. The necessity for several attempts is not unusual, but it is unusual to see backflow of blood in this technique. Repeated failure should lead to cessation of effort rather than dogged persistence with a blind technique in an area fraught with potential hazards.

If the Intracath moves forward easily through the needle, it can be assumed that the catheter is probably within a large vessel. After full insertion, the needle guard is put in place, and tape is applied over the needle guard to secure it to the skin. In addition, a small gauze dressing dipped in antiseptic solution is applied around the point where the Intracath passes through the skin. A suitable intravenous bottle is attached via a three-way stopcock to the subclavian line and the bottle dropped below the level of the patient. A back flush of blood into the tubing at this point indicates that the line is in a large vein or the right atrium. The final dressing of the wound now takes place, and the last 4 or 5 cm of the polyethylene line should be taped so that this length of the catheter is completely sealed off from the outside. Radiologic confirmation of the position of the catheter is useful, because misdirection of the tip into the external jugular vein or opposite subclavian vein is an occasional problem. The x-ray can also delineate any pneumothorax or hemothorax that may have occurred. Having the patient rotate his face toward the operator during insertion will narrow the angle of the jugular-subclavian vein junction and lessen the chance of catheterizing the jugular vein.

If the line is to be used for hyperalimentation, a regular

and strict cleansing of the catheter skin junction must be performed to prevent septic complications. Every 48 hours, the dressings are removed under sterile precaution, and the skin site carefully cleansed with a suitable antiseptic solution. In addition, the catheter is withdrawn slightly, cleansed with alcohol, then readvanced. It is not usually necessary to suture the catheter in place, but this is an added safety feature. The use of a Millipore filter in the hyperalimentation line is also an essential contamination precaution. Reported complications of this procedure include pneumothorax, mediastinal bleeding, hemothorax, venous thrombosis, brachial plexus injury, air embolism, thoracic duct injury, pericardial tamponade, cardiac arrhythmias, cardiac perforation, and catheter-induced sepsis. With the technique described, most of these complications can be avoided, particularly if undue persistence is avoided when the technique appears difficult. An inadvertent subclavian artery puncture is often unrecognized; even if it is detected, the position of the artery behind the clavicle makes compression difficult. However, encircling the clavicle with thumb and forefinger at the presumed site of injury and squeezing will frequently stop the bleeding.

An alternative technique, and probably the more standard one, is to attach a syringe to the Intracath catheter. Aspiration on this syringe, when the needle is felt to be within the lumen of the subclavian vein, will produce a back flush of venous blood. This modification affords reassurance that the catheter tip is in the proper position, and also avoids the theoretical hazard of shearing off the polyethylene tubing if withdrawal of the catheter into the needle is necessary for a second pass. However, opening the catheter to attach a syringe exposes the line to potential contamination; gloves and probably a mask should be worn if this modification is chosen. Also, a wider field should be cleansed and towel drapes should be used to avoid potential soiling of the exposed polyethylene line. For those without great experience in the technique of subclavian vein catheterization, a no. 22 spinal needle attached to a syringe may be used to locate the vein prior to passage of the larger Intracath needle. The return of blood of venous coloration will correctly localize the vessel, and should the artery be inadvertently entered, the small size of the needle will obviate serious bleeding. The no. 22 spinal needle with syringe attached may even be introduced through the lumen of the larger Intracath, and when proper position is indicated by venous blood return into the syringe, the Intracath may be slid forward over the spinal needle in a modification of the Seldinger wire technique. The spinal needle is then withdrawn from the Intracath, the syringe reattached to the Intracath hub, and aspiration is repeated to confirm proper location before passage of the polyethylene tubing.

Catheter-induced sepsis remains a problem, particularly with hyperalimentation lines. Unexplained septic episodes should lead to a prompt removal of any indwelling venous lines. Although the source of sepsis frequently will be proved to be elsewhere, the consequences of making this assumption incorrectly warrant a conservative approach.

2.5. SWAN-GANZ CATHETER PLACEMENT

The bedside placement of a flow-directed or Swan-Ganz catheter for the measurement of pulmonary capillary wedge pressure has proved a valuable adjunct in the management of myocardial infarction, preoperative and postoperative cardiac patients, and other individuals with suspected central pump failure. Two techniques will be discussed for the insertion of this catheter.

MATERIAL
A sterile venous cutdown set (see Section 2.6, Venous Cutdowns), Swan-Ganz catheter set. Floor supplies: intravenous solution and tubing, antiseptic solution, tape, pressure recording transducer, and electrocardiograph machine.

Even though passage of this catheter is slightly facilitated by fluoroscopic monitoring, blind passage is successful in a high percentage of cases and permits bedside insertion of the unit. The Swan-Ganz catheter is an extruded polyvinylchloride catheter of no. 5 or no. 7 French outer diameter, constructed with a latex balloon fastened one millimeter from the tip and connected via a side hole in the shaft to a small lumen parallel to the major lumen. The balloon is normally inflated to a volume of 0.8 ml and has a bursting volume of 3 ml. A syringe is attached to a special stopcock which connects the distal end of the catheter to the small lumen, and the balloon should be checked for integrity before insertion.

TECHNIQUE

1. The major lumen is connected to a pressure monitor and the catheter is introduced via an antecubital, basilic vein cutdown (see Section 2.6, Venous Cutdowns).

Although this complication is unusual, passage of the catheter through the heart is on occasion associated with premature ventricular contractions, and the patient should have a monitoring electrocardiograph during passage. The premature ventricular contractions are usually encountered as the catheter passes the tricuspid valve. It is also prudent to have a defibrillator and intravenous lidocaine solution on standby availability. The catheter is advanced 35 cm. Difficulty in passage of the catheter across the axilla may be facilitated by manipulating the arm (see section 2.6, Venous Cutdowns), or by inflating the balloon with 0.4 to 0.6 ml of air, then withdrawing the catheter slightly before readvancement. As the catheter enters the thorax, a cough will produce 40 mm or more deflection in the pressure tracing. A typical pressure tracing seen as the catheter passes from the right atrium to the right ventricle and subsequently into the pulmonary artery is illustrated by Figure 2.8. The balloon is now inflated to a total of 0.8 ml. If more than 15 cm of the catheter is advanced into the right ventricle without recording a pulmonary artery pressure, the catheter is in all likelihood doubled up in the ventricle; it should be withdrawn to the atrium and passage begun anew. After inflation, the catheter is allowed to bounce from the right ventricle into the pulmonary artery and to proceed downstream until a pressure resembling pulmonary artery wedge pressure is obtained (see Figure 2.8). At this point, the balloon is deflated, and pulmonary artery-type pressure readings should be seen again. The catheter is now advanced

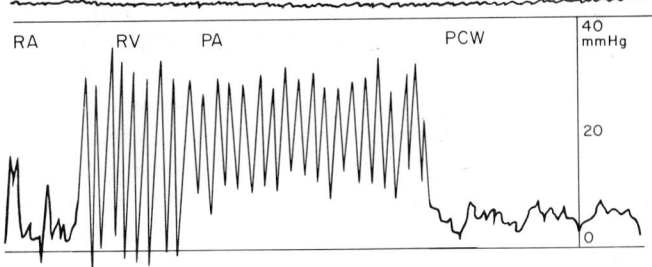

Figure 2.8.

Idealized but typical pressure tracings seen during advancement of a Swan-Ganz catheter. **RA**: right atrial tracing; **RV**: right ventricular tracing; **PA**: pulmonary artery tracing (note increased diastolic pressure); **PCW**: pulmonary capillary wedge tracing.

into the wedge position by moving it forward another 1 to 3 cm. When wedge pressure is required, the catheter balloon is inflated without further manipulation.

Minimal motion artifact characterizes this system. Before each filling of the balloon for wedge pressure, the syringe should be disconnected from the adapter and reconnected, to assure a neutral position of the balloon before inflation. If any chance exists that the catheter may pass into the left side of the heart, carbon dioxide should be used to fill the balloon. Overdistension of the balloon will give artifactual readings and should be avoided. With balloon inflation, arterialized blood should be returned (i.e., left heart blood) and can be used as a check on proper wedge position. The catheter is secured as described in the section on Venous Cutdowns and the wound closed (see section 2.6).

In approximately 5 percent of patients, the balloon will either not pass out of the heart or not wedge properly. These are individuals usually with valvular disease, and in particular, pulmonary artery hypertension. In this latter case, wedging is often difficult, and this is an instance where portable fluoroscopy can be of assistance. Nevertheless, the ability to obtain pulmonary artery pressure, even without pulmonary capillary wedge pressures, can yield valuable diagnostic information. The use of this catheter is on rare occasion associated with pulmonary infarcts. As is true with any indwelling central line, the potential for infection is also a recognized hazard, and warrants meticulous wound care (see section 2.6).

Currently, these catheters may be obtained with an additional lumen for the measurement of cardiac output. However, the basic technique for insertion is the same.

2. An alternative method for passing the catheter into the right atrium is via the internal jugular vein (generally the right-sided vein), using the Cournand technique.

The short and direct route from the internal jugular vein to the right atrium eases passage, and the Cournand technique enables the catheter to be passed without necessity for a cutdown. To introduce the Swan-Ganz catheter via this route, a Cournand wire introducing kit will be necessary, such as the Desilets-Hoffman Introducer, made by the U.S.C.I. Division of Bard. This consists of a Cournand wire, approximately 35 cm long, and an inner and an outer sleeve, the latter with a Luer-Lok adapter. The introducer must be at least one French size larger than the catheter to be passed through it.

The patient is positioned in the Trendelenburg position with the face turned away from the side to be used. The skin of the neck is prepared widely, and gloves are worn. The posterior edge of the sternocleidomastoid muscle is traced out, and the site for insertion is chosen either where a fairly constant branch of the external jugular crosses the posterior border of this muscle or at a site one-half of the way between the clavicular head of the muscle and its attachment to the mastoid process. Xylocaine is infiltrated at this site and, to ease passage of the Cournand wire and sleeves, a small nick is made here with a no. 11 scalpel blade. It is first ascertained that the vein can be aspirated by introducing a no. 23 spinal needle attached to a syringe through this nick, at a 45 degree angle to the skin, passing the needle parallel to the posterior border of the sternocleidomastoid muscle, aiming between the clavicular and sternal heads of the sternocleidomastoid muscle (Figure 2.9). Care should be taken to avoid the carotid artery, which is within the same vascular sheath. The pulsations of this artery can often be felt against the needle tip if it is off

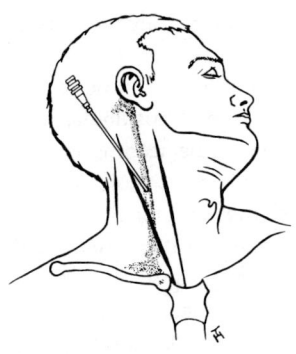

Figure 2.9.

Internal jugular vein puncture for passage of a Swan-Ganz catheter. Note that the skin puncture site is approximately half way between the clavicular and the mastoid attachments of the sternocleidomastoid muscle.

course. The needle is withdrawn to a subcutaneous position and redirected. Free aspiration of venous blood indicates that the vein has been located. The spinal needle is now removed and a 16-gauge plastic Rochester-type needle (such as the Angiocath) is now used to follow this path and puncture the vein. This size catheter will accommodate the Cournand wire of the no. 8 French introducer set. When blood is once again freely returned into a syringe attached to the Rochester needle, the inner metal needle is withdrawn, leaving the catheter in place in the vein. It is important to use a plastic catheter of this kind, because a needle left in the vein on withdrawal might shear off the Cournand wire. The wire is advanced through the Angiocath and the latter is removed. The inner jacket is now advanced over the wire into the jugular vein and the wire is removed. The outer jacket is advanced its full length over the inner jacket and the inner jacket is removed. This outer jacket will now accommodate the proper sized French Swan-Ganz catheter, which is passed with the same electrocardiographic and pressure monitoring precautions described above. When the catheter is in satisfactory position, the outer sleeve is withdrawn from the skin, but remains around the catheter. The Swan-Ganz catheter itself is stitched to the skin and a single stitch is used to close the nick. An antibiotic ointment may be applied around the entry point. The catheter is securely taped to the neck and looped so as to allow the patient comfortable motion. Properly secured, the transjugular route allows stable catheter placement to be accomplished. Regardless of the route chosen, a chest x-ray should be taken to confirm proper location of the catheter tip.

Prior to insertion of the catheter, the monitor unit should be properly calibrated and all lines to the transducer cleared of bubbles, which will cause damping of the pulmonary artery wave form. Once the catheter is in place and connected, the transducer should be placed at the level of the right atrium and the lines flushed again of any bubbles prior to making the first reading. Should the patient's position with relation to the transducer be changed, as in sitting up, the transducer must also be repositioned in its proper relationship to the right atrium, to continue accurate recording.

2.6. VENOUS CUTDOWNS

The ability to perform a rapid and secure venous cutdown can, in emergency situations, be a life-saving technique. Although this is strictly speaking a "surgical" procedure, it is so simple, and the need for it is so likely to arise when no surgeon is immediately available, that skill in its performance should be mastered by every physician with clinical responsibilities.

Although subclavian vein catheterization is more rapidly accomplished and has in large measure replaced venous cutdowns, this is a prime example of surgical fadism; the skills acquired performing cutdowns are lost to the detriment of the patient. Distal venous cutdowns are still indicated when central venous pressure measurements are not required, and cutdowns are generally safer and more stable than subclavian catheterization, because they are performed under direct vision.

Indications for a cutdown are many, and include administration of therapeutic fluids during shock or cardiac resuscitation, monitoring of central venous pressure, rapid and massive blood transfusions, administration of locally toxic or hypertonic fluids, when intravenous therapy will be prolonged, or when peripheral veins are unsuitable for standard venous infusions.

The technique to be described is applicable for venous cutdowns wherever done, but there are peculiarities for each individual location, and knowledge of them will be of assistance in making the proper choice. There are five common sites for venous cutdowns. (While technically feasible, the tendency of catheters in the femoral vein to throw emboli makes this area undesirable, and this location will not be discussed. Children tolerate cannulation of this vessel better than adults, and central venous lines into the femoral vein by way of the greater saphenous vein are commonly employed during major surgery. This procedure usually requires general anesthesia, however, and it is not a bedside procedure.)

Saphenous Vein at the Ankle

The saphenous vein as it crosses in front of the medial malleolus is a constant and large vessel, easily reached through a short horizontal incision 2 cm above and 1 cm anterior to the point of greatest bulge of the malleolus. *It is the vein of choice when time is essential,* as in cardiac arrest and resuscitation. Carry dissection rapidly down to the periosteum; the vein will invariably lie anterior at this point and may quickly be brought into the incision by sweeping a curved hemostat anteriorly, then superficially from the bone (Figure 2.10). There are no other important structures in this area, although an inconsequential terminal twig of the saphenous nerve may accompany the vein. A catheter here will not measure central venous pressure because of the saphenous valves, and blood samples cannot be aspirated for the same reason. Therefore, there should be no compulsion to run in the line for more than 2 or 3 cm (and less in infants). When used in infants, it will be necessary to immobilize the ankle by firmly taping both the foot and lower leg to a padded board, with an extra sponge between the board and the lateral malleolus. Early phlebitis here is often associated with catheters pushed in an inordinate length. Regardless of technique, however, a superficial phlebitis occurs regularly after 48 hours, and it may be severe if pressor drugs are given in this area. For this reason, the use of the saphenous cutdown should be limited to emergency situations and when infusions will not be prolonged.

Cephalic Vein at the Wrist

This useful vessel is too often overlooked. It may be rapidly and easily reached in its superficial location on the radial side of the wrist through a 2-cm horizontal incision, directly over the radial styloid and midway between the dorsal and volar surfaces of the wrist. The vein is large enough to accept either a catheter or beaded needle, and next to the saphenous vein it is the most accessible large vein in the body. When a central venous line is not required, and when the saphenous vein cutdown is not suitable, this constant vessel makes an excellent second choice. The wrist should be stabilized on a handboard after placement of this line.

Basilic Vein in the Antecubital Space

This vein, or venous system, is most frequently selected when it is desired to run the catheter into the subclavian vein or more centrally to monitor venous pressure. Because they are not subject to embolism formation as readily, and because intra-abdominal pressures often give erroneous venous pressure measurements, central venous catheters led in by upper extremity veins are almost uniformly preferable to those led in by veins in the legs. A technique for blind cannulation of the subclavian vein is described in Section 2.3, Intravenous Infusions.

    A common mistake is to make the horizontal incision directly over the antecubital space or its lateral aspect. This makes it likely that the catheter will be introduced into a tributary of the cephalic system rather than of the basilic system; it is almost impossible to enter the subclavian vein when the cephalic vein is cannulated at this level. To avoid this problem, make the incision 3 cm proximal to the ante-

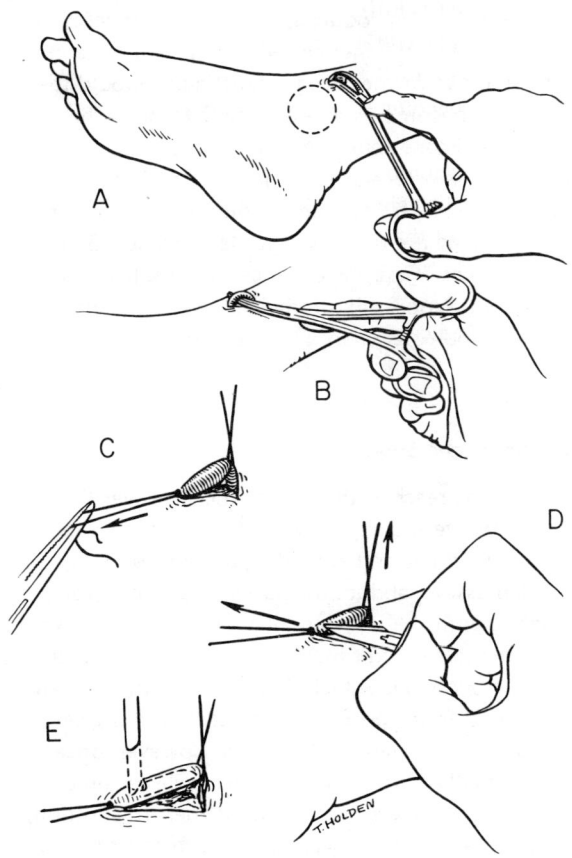

Figure 2.10.

Saphenous vein cutdown. (**A, B**) Vein is bluntly dissected free with a hemostat and swept forward from the medial malleolus into the incision. (**C**) Method of holding ligated vein. (**D**) Venotomy—the no. 11 blade, with the blade up, is passed horizontally through the vessel. (**E**) Catheter is introduced through venotomy at right angles to vessel wall before redirecting tip forward.

cubital space and well around on the inner aspect of the arm. Remember that large and useful veins may lie immediately beneath the skin here, and care should be taken not to sever them with the skin incision. In addition, the veins accompanying the brachial artery may be used if the basilic vessel cannot be located.

Once the catheter is introduced, advance it as quickly as possible. Its presence will induce venospasm rapidly, and if delayed it will make further progress difficult. Should the catheter seem to become stuck as it passes through the axilla, have an assistant abduct the arm while rotating the catheter between thumb and forefinger. This will often straighten the basilic vein as it enters the axillary vein, and alter the position of the tip so that it may advance. Some doctors prefer to estimate the distance to the subclavian vein, and then tie a loose silk on the catheter that length from the tip, to indicate when it has been run in the proper distance.

Cephalic Vein on the Shoulder

This vessel may be reached through an incision over the deltopectoral groove and parallel with it, commencing about 1 cm below the clavicle and extending distally for 3 cm. To locate this depression, abduct the patient's arm passively while palpating with the free hand immediately medial to the coracoid process. In this manner, it may be accurately felt even in the obese individual. At this point, the cephalic vein lies deep within the groove, and dissection must be carried a little further than at other sites. However, once isolated, it is usually quite easy from this angle to run a catheter into the subclavian vessel and further. In addition, cutdowns here are peculiarly free of the problems of early phlebitis that plague other sites, and high cephalic cutdowns can function beautifully for over two weeks. They also allow the patient free use of the arm. Thus, when time is not pressing, and extended use is likely, as in the patient with a severe stroke, this site offers distinct advantages over the antecubital space. Figure 2.11 illustrates the proper location for cutdown incisions in the upper extremity.

The External Jugular Vein

Although it is possible to isolate and cannulate this vein, its tortuous course often makes it difficult to enter the catheter into the subclavian vein, and its location is not favorable

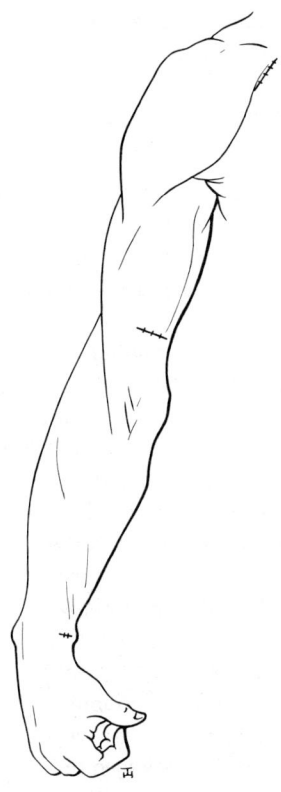

Figure 2.11.

Three common sites for venous cutdowns in the upper extremity. Antecubital incision is above the elbow crease and on the inner aspect of the arm.

for stabilization of the line, once in place. It should not be tried during cardiac resuscitation—there is no room to work. To locate the vein, extend the neck by placing a pillow beneath the patient's shoulders, and have him turn his face away from the selected side. Press in firmly with the full length of the index finger directly above the clavicle, compressing the vein at this point. A 2-cm horizontal incision immediately over the vessel and about 3 fingerbreadths above the clavicle is proper. A cutdown here should be used when arm veins have proved unfeasible. When a short central venous line such as a high cephalic cutdown or external jugular vein cutdown is used, the potential for air embolism exists if the intravenous tubing and catheter adapter become disconnected. All junctions must be firmly taped together and taped securely to the patient.

MATERIAL

A sterile cutdown set, containing scalpel handle, nos. 15 and 11 blades, small vascular scissors with sharp tips, suture scissors, small, curved dissection scissors, two curved hemostats, two curved mosquito hemostats, fine-toothed (vascular) and regular-toothed forceps, small self-retaining retractor, 5-ml syringe, 25-gauge and 22-gauge needles, 4 sterile towels, sterile sponges, 4–0 skin silks with straight needles, ampules of local anesthetic. Floor supplies: suitable packaged catheter of polyethylene or Silastic, blunt-ended needle (if catheter does not come with an attached female adapter for the intravenous tubing), intravenous solution and tubing, with a central venous pressure set if desired, antiseptic solution, tape (1 inch wide and torn in many 3-inch strips).

Comment. Good lighting is a must; to attempt a cutdown, particularly in the upper extremity, without adequate lighting is to court frustration and failure. A central venous pressure set now is available as a complete packaged unit with a three-way stopcock and manometer (Fenwal), and may readily be adapted to use with standard intravenous infusion sets.

Intracath units containing 24-inch catheters with wire stylets are available for the percutaneous placement of central venous pressure lines. When large vessels of the basilic system are visible, these units are suitable alternatives to a cutdown. The directions with the unit should be followed explicitly, particularly the cautions regarding the use of the bevel cover to prevent shearing of the catheter by the needle tip. The puncture site should also be protected with a separate sterile dressing.

TECHNIQUE

Figure 2.10 illustrates the ankle cutdown, but the technique is the same for all locations. Hands are washed, and mask, sterile gown, and gloves worn. For a wrist or antecubital space cutdown, place the patient's arm in an abducted position for ease of access. Externally rotate the ankle as much as possible for a saphenous cutdown. Cleanse and drape the area selected, infiltrate a local anesthetic along the projected line of incision, and make the skin incision suggested. Once through the skin, deep dissection should be blunt, and the jaws of the curved hemostat spread parallel with the long axis of the vein, to disclose it and dissect it free. A tourniquet around the arm and leg may help to pinpoint the location of the vessel, but be sure to remove it before incising into the wall. A vein distended with blood is easy enough to identify, but in its normal state it will appear more white than blue. It has a characteristically elastic feel and tubular shape, however, that will assist in identification. Several veins may be seen during the dissection, particularly in the antecubital area, but do not waste effort over vessels too small to allow passage of the catheter. A small vein may be stretched enough to introduce the cannula, but venospasm will defeat efforts to advance it. A good rule of thumb is not to select any vein whose outside diameter undistended is less than two-thirds that of the catheter.

Pass a 4-0 silk beneath the vein as distal as possible, and using this as a retractor to bring the vessel into the incision, bluntly clear it of surrounding tissue with the tips of the hemostat. This important step affords a good idea of the true size of the vein. Free at least a 2-cm length of vein, then pass another silk beneath it at the proximal end of the dissection. Tie down the distal silk and use the weight of an attached hemostat to maintain tension on this ligature along the long axis of the vein. If necessary, clip the hemostat to both silk and towel to keep the ligature taut; this is the only way to keep the vessel straight and up in the incision, short of the luxury of an assistant.

Cut the tip of the catheter on a slight bevel to aid in introducing it into the vein, but if it is a polyethylene catheter and somewhat stiff, snip off the tiny pointed tip of this beveled end to prevent it from puncturing the vessel wall as it advances. Fill the catheter with saline solution and leave the syringe attached. For infants, polyethylene catheters may be stretched lengthwise at their tips, thus narrowing them and easing their introduction and passage.

Select a site near the distal ligature to open the vein. Many methods are used in making a venotomy, and certainly a simple full-thickness cut made halfway through the vein with the sharp vascular scissors will ordinarily be adequate. However, to avoid cutting too deeply into the vein or transecting it completely, the use of the no. 11 scalpel blade is useful. Do not mount the blade on a handle, but pick it up with the blade facing up, as shown in Figure 2.10. Lightly hold up on the proximal silk to control back-bleeding, and select a depth on the vein that will transect about one-half its diameter. Place the tip of the blade at this point, and pass it horizontally through the vessel. Inasmuch as the blade will cut only upward and is under direct vision, it will be difficult to cut too deeply. This is an exceptionally useful trick in pediatric cutdowns, where vessels are tiny and the chances of inadvertent transection correspondingly great. The venotomy may be stretched by introducing the tips of the mosquito hemostat and gently opening them.

The tip of the catheter is now introduced by first pressing it through the opening, against the vessel wall opposite, before changing the direction of the thrust to one paralleling the long axis of the vein and threading the cannula forward. Should this initial step prove difficult, the proximal lip of the venotomy may be grasped with the vascular forceps to supply countertraction. While advancing the catheter, maintain vessel tension by light traction on the distal ligature.

The length of catheter passed into the vein will be dictated by the anatomic position of the vessel and purpose of the cutdown, as described earlier. When it is advanced a satisfactory length, tie down the proximal ligature around vein and catheter, taking care not to occlude the latter by tying it too tightly. This procedure will prevent leakage, but it should not be relied upon to keep the catheter in the vein. The position of a central venous line without a radiopaque marker may be checked simply by filling the catheter with

Hypaque solution, clamping it, and having an appropriate x-ray taken.

Close the skin with interrupted silks (it is not necessary or desirable to anchor the line at the skin level with a silk stitch, for it may pinch the lumen), and apply a dry, small dressing secured with several of the short pretorn tape strips. Some advise running a long strip of adhesive around the catheter from the dressing to its hub to avoid inadvertent dislodgment. The line may be adequately anchored simply by taping it to the extremity with two short strips at some distance from the dressing; this has the advantage of conserving the catheter's natural pliability and prevents the kinking often caused by the long tape strips.

The manometer for a central venous pressure line should be fixed to a suitable rigid structure, such as an intravenous pole, and the zero point on the water level set at the level of the mid-right atrium, with the patient in a supine position on a flat bed. A carpenter's level should be used, taking as a landmark the sternal prominence at the second intercostal space, the angle of Louis. The level is placed at a point on the patient's lateral thoracic wall approximately 5 cm below this sternal angle, and the manometer marked where the level crosses it when the measuring bubble is in the center of the gauge. Inaccurate location of this zero point in relationship to the patient's mid-right atrial level is one of the common causes for inaccurate central venous pressure readings. Other problems leading to inaccuracy with upper extremity central venous pressure lines are obstruction of the catheter tip against the side wall of the vein, or ball-valve obstruction at the catheter tip by clot, giving false low readings. Often withdrawal of the catheter tip a few millimeters will correct the problem arising when the tip is against the vein wall.

Before a central venous line is taped in place permanently, it should be seen that the central venous pressure line is functioning adequately. This is best gauged by the presence of normal respiratory variations in the central venous pressure. Hyperventilation will cause low readings if the fluid level in the manometer does not have time to rise back up to the true venous pressure between respirations. Also, coughing or straining during measurement will raise the central venous pressure transiently. If the catheter has not been passed into the central venous system, or if it is inadvertently passed into the right ventricle, the readings will be inaccurate or unobtainable. Right ventricular placement might be suspected if the manometer fluctuations are violent, and the position of the line should be checked radiologically.

Indwelling venous lines have been implicated as sources of septicemia, *and any cutdown should be looked upon with suspicion if the patient is running an unexplained septic course.* A strict aseptic technique, antibiotic jelly applied at the catheter-skin junction, and frequent dressing changes offer partial protection. The extremity carrying the venous line should be checked twice daily for the appearance of phlebitis, and worrisome catheters should be removed at once and cultured.

2.7. ARTERIAL CUTDOWNS

An arterial catheter for the accurate and continuous measurement of blood pressure has become increasingly important as new techniques and treatments for which the standard blood pressure cuff is totally inadequate become common practice. These include cardiopulmonary bypass, the treatment of profound shock with or without vasodilatory drugs, clinical crisis patients of many types, and postresuscitation monitoring and pressure monitoring during surgery in which large volumes of blood are routinely needed, such as aortic aneurysm resections. Although arterial pressures may be measured from such a line by as simple a gauge as a balanced U-shaped mercury manometer, the increasing sophistication of bedside monitors allows the physician a wide choice of transducer-mediated equipment for continuous pressure recording. Often it is neither practical nor desirable to move a patient to the operating room for placement of such a catheter, and such a move is not necessary. The insertion of a line into the radial artery is no more difficult than the insertion of a central venous catheter, and the two are often needed together, the observation of central venous pressure being of equal importance in all the conditions described above. Section 2.6, Venous Cutdowns, should be reviewed, for it will be referred to later.

By anatomic dissection, there are rare individuals in whom the anastomoses between the ulnar and radial vasculature in the palmar arches are small or absent. Theoretically, interruption of the radial supply by a catheter in these people could lead to severe ischemia on the radial side of the hand. In practice, however, the tiny fraction of patients who do develop real problems with peripheral supply are those with severe reduction in central cardiac output, regardless of their distal vascular anatomy. If the situation permits, one should perform the Allen test to assess the existence of open channels between radial and ulnar circuits. In this test, the patient makes a tight fist, and while the hand is clenched, the radial and ulnar arteries are occluded. When the hand is opened, the ulnar vessel is released, and the hand is inspected for return of color while firm pressure is maintained on the radial pulse. Flushing of the entire hand is considered presumptive evidence of adequate ulnar collateral blood supply. If the hand fails to blush throughout until the radial artery is released, the cutdown site should be moved higher in the forearm to protect distal radial-ulnar anastomoses in muscles and via vessels running along the interosseous membrane. This test should not be interpreted as an absolute contraindication to the use of an arterial catheter, and it is worthless in the presence of shock.

MATERIAL

The equipment and preparation required are precisely the same as those for venous cutdowns (see Section 2.6), with the addition of a Rochester-type needle with a flaring collar, such as the Argyle 16-gauge, 2-inch Medicut cannula, a package of 3–0 silk on a cutting needle, and a French-eye needle. Again, the need for proper lighting is needed.

TECHNIQUE

The operator should wash thoroughly and wear gloves and mask, and preferably a gown. The arm is placed on a board or bedside stand for access, and cleansed from hand to antecubital space. After infiltration with a local anesthetic (*no epinephrine*), a vertical incision is made directly over the radial pulse at the wrist, or over its rarely palpable deep location in the midforearm. The vessel lies beneath the bulk of the brachioradialis muscle at this higher spot, and a longer incision must be used to reach it with adequate exposure. In addition, its location here is only about 1 cm lateral to midline, and care should be taken not to make the incision too far to the radial side.

The cannula is first prepared by passing a single 3-0 silk through a circular piece of sterile Silastic or rubber tubing previously pushed up over the flare of the collar. In the absence of a suitable sleeve, this stitch may be driven through the Medicut itself far enough distally on the collar to be sealed when the extension tubing is in place. Cut boldly for the pulse until the artery, with its characteristic white, pulsatile, absolutely round appearance and elastic feel, is identified. Two venae comitantes accompany the artery throughout its course, and the radial nerve lies lateral to it in the forearm.

Dissect the vessel free with a curved hemostat for a length of 2 cm and bring it up into the incision with an encircling but untied 4-0 silk. A very small arteriotomy is made with a vascular scissors or no. 11 blade (see Section 2.6), while maintaining proximal control with the silk. The cannula may also be introduced by direct puncture, as illustrated (Figure 2.12A). Insert the Medicut cannula through the opening, remove the inner needle, and attach a clamped saline-filled length of extension tubing such as the Plexitron R33 Anesthesia Extension Set (Baxter). Now run in the outer sleeve until its flaring collar fits snugly into the arteriotomy and prevents leakage.

To hold the cannula in this position against an arterial pulse, the preplaced stitch is run out both sides of the proximal end of the incision, using the French needle, and

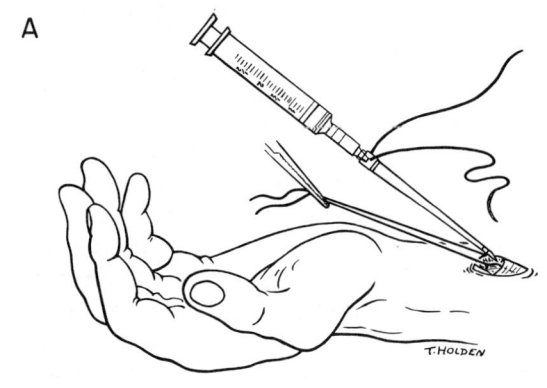

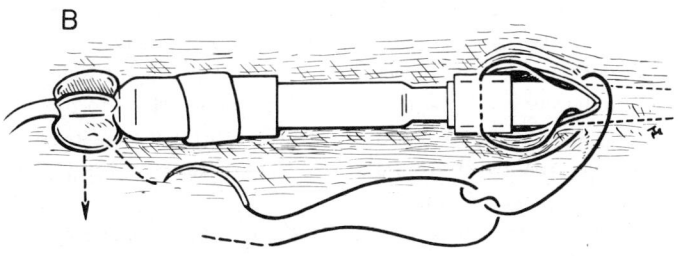

Figure 2.12.
"No ligature" method of introducing a radial artery catheter. (**A**) Direct puncture of artery using Argyle Medicut cannula. Note structure through improvised collar around cannula. (**B**) Stabilization of cannula—suture passes from inside to outside of distal end of the incision, is next tied (holding cannula in artery), then passes through plastic wings on I.V. tubing, and is tied again (holding tubing in cannula). No deep ligatures are required.

is tied under slight tension. The extension tubing is secured to the cannula by the same stitch passing through any solid piece of plastic molding near the end of the extension set and the collar (Figure 2.12B). After flushing the catheter free with a small amount of heparinized saline solution, the incision is closed with a single layer of 4-0 silk skin stitches, a bactericidal jelly is layered around the cannula, and a dry dressing is applied. The hand is secured to a board, and the tubing is looped and taped, as illustrated by Figure 2.6, to protect the line against an inadvertent tug.

An arterial line of PE 190 or 200 polyethylene, fitted with a blunt needle, may also be run in the artery for 2 cm in precisely the same manner as described for venous cutdowns, ligating the artery distally and holding the catheter in place with a cinching ligature around both vessel and cannula proximally. The method first described, however, has the following advantages. (1) Because no ligature is left around the artery, many patients will have a good return of pulse following removal of the cannula. (2) A distal ligature forms an obstruction that often makes it necessary to reopen the incision to ligate the artery for bleeding when the polyethylene catheter is removed. With distal runoff present, a Medicut cannula can usually be removed simply by cutting the single stitch and applying 5 minutes of firm pressure over the artery after it is pulled out. If a polyethylene line is used, leave a stitch passing through tissue immediately proximal to the arteriotomy and deep to the artery so that the long ends, protruding through the closed incision, may be knotted and tied down after removal of the catheter to gain hemostasis.

In many hospitals, a formal arterial cutdown has been replaced by direct needle puncture of the artery, using a medium bore Rochester-type needle such as the 18-gauge, 2-inch Angiocath. This is an acceptable alternative technique if the patient has a palpable radial pulse.

The wrist is hyperextended over a small towel roll and taped to a handboard. A small wheal of anesthetic may be placed where the needle puncture for the arterial line is planned. The puncture site should be approximately at the same position that an incision would be made for an arterial cutdown. The Angiocath needle is introduced at a 45-degree angle, with the bevel up. No syringe is attached to the needle, and any plug is removed from its back end, so that blood will run freely when the artery is punctured. The puncture site should be directly over the radial pulse, and the course of the needle should be directed straight for the artery until arterial blood freely flows from the rear of the

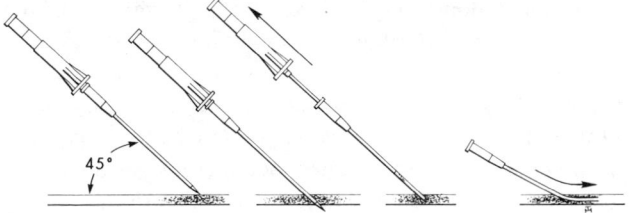

Figure 2.13.

Radial artery puncture. Note proper angle of approach to artery, and that needle tip actually penetrates posterior wall of the vessel, to ensure proper intraluminal position of the shorter catheter. The needle is then withdrawn and the catheter advanced with the hub of the tubing at less of an angle to the long axis of the vessel.

Angiocath (Figure 2.13). Once blood appears, the needle is advanced a few millimeters more on its original course until no further blood is seen. The needle point has now transected the artery and lies beyond the lumen, while the end of the Teflon catheter, situated slightly distal to the point of the steel needle, is within the lumen of the artery. The steel needle is withdrawn approximately 5 mm so that it no longer protrudes past the end of the Teflon catheter. The catheter and needle are next withdrawn very slightly, together as a unit, until blood once again begins to well out from the hub of the catheter. At this point, it is assumed that the tip of the Teflon catheter is lying free in the lumen of the radial artery and is not up against a wall. The entire unit is now depressed, so that the angle with the skin is more like 30 than 45 degrees, and the needle and catheter are slowly advanced together into the artery, approximately a distance of 2 to 3 cm. The steel needle is left within the lumen of the Teflon catheter during this advancement, for the added stiffness makes passage easier. However, some prefer to remove the steel needle completely before advancing the Teflon catheter. While the needle is moving forward, blood should be freely welling from the hub of the catheter at all times. This assures the operator that the catheter is within the lumen of the vessel. Once adequate length is run in, the steel needle is removed completely and a three-way stopcock and monitoring line are attached to the hub of the Teflon catheter. The catheter and the three-way stopcock are firmly taped together, the roll is removed from behind the patient's wrist, and the radial artery unit is firmly taped to the wrist. The wrist and hand are also taped in a neutral, but supinated, position on a handboard as long as the radial artery line is in use. Careful nursing attention to the adequate taping of this unit is necessary, for accidental dislodgement of the three-way stopcock from the Teflon catheter or the monitoring line from the stopcock can lead to considerable hemorrhage.

Such a line, filled with heparosaline solution, may now be directly connected to the pressure monitoring device. It is advisable to flush the line about every 4 hours with a few milliliters of heparosaline solution. Despite the most meticulous care, some damping of the arterial pressure is noted usually by 48 to 72 hours, and 96 hours is about the normal life of most arterial lines. Line life may be extended by incorporating a pressurized delivery system that allows continuous rather than intermittent infusion of dilute heparosaline solution into the artery. One such unit is called Intraflo, manufactured by Sorenson Research. If mottling of the skin of the fingers or hand occurs at any time, the catheter must be removed at once.

3.

ASPIRATION TECHNIQUES

3.1. THORACENTESIS

The nature of the intrathoracic fluid to be drained will usually indicate the proper approach to thoracentesis. Certainly the technique is not applicable for the automobile accident or gunshot victim with an acute, massive hemothorax, nor is it sufficient to handle most empyemas except for diagnosis and cultures. But even when clearly indicated, success in removal of fluid will most consistently be obtained by the doctor who has first localized the fluid accurately through careful physical examination and chest x-rays (at least P-A and lateral views, and obliques if possible). It is only with this information that the proper anatomic approach to loculated fluid is assured; it should precede every thoracentesis.

The goals of thoracentesis are three: diagnosis, therapy, and prophylaxis. Diagnostic taps are uniformly indicated whenever there is a pleural effusion of unknown etiology. Therapeutic thoracenteses are used in the treatment of congestive heart failure, malignancy (with the option of instilling antitumor agents through the same needle), postoperative patients on the cardiovascular and thoracic services, and many others. In these patients, removal of the fluid mantle surrounding the lung often results in dramatically improved pulmonary function. By "prophylaxis" is meant the eradication of undrained pockets of fluid, even small ones, whenever feasible, in the knowledge that pleural fluid, particularly when loculated, has the potential for abscess formation. Because one route by which infection can be introduced is via the thoracentesis needle, strict aseptic technique is essential.

MATERIAL

Sterile thoracentesis kit: 50-ml syringe with Luer-Lok adapter, two 10-ml syringes, disposable 25-gauge, 20-gauge, and 18-gauge needles, 17-gauge and 15-gauge short-beveled needles of 3-inch length, Kelly clamp, culture tubes with stoppers, three-way stopcock with a 10-inch length of tubing attached to the side arm, no. 11 blade, 2 ampules of local anesthetic, 4 sterile towels, dry sponges. Commercial thoracentesis kits are also widely available. Floor supplies: heparin, evacuated thoracentesis flask or open-topped liter jugs, antiseptic-soaked sponges, and sterile gloves.

Comment. Many physicians have successfully used the large-bore 14-gauge, 2-inch Intracath for thoracentesis, attaching the three-way stopcock to the catheter after withdrawing the needle from the chest wall. There is no question that this is a satisfactory instrument and that the danger of lung injury is lessened without the needle. It does have several disadvantages: drainage is slower, the catheter will become more easily plugged with fibrin or clots, and it is difficult to redirect the tip with any accuracy.

TECHNIQUE

Large, nonloculated pleural effusions are most easily drained through the fifth or sixth intercostal space in the midaxillary line. The patient is in bed, head up about 60 degrees, and with his back supported. The arm on the side to be tapped is held over the head, grasped by the other hand, if necessary, for support (Figure 3.1). This position is also proper for the occasional anterior thoracentesis, done for isolated anterior collections, usually through the third or

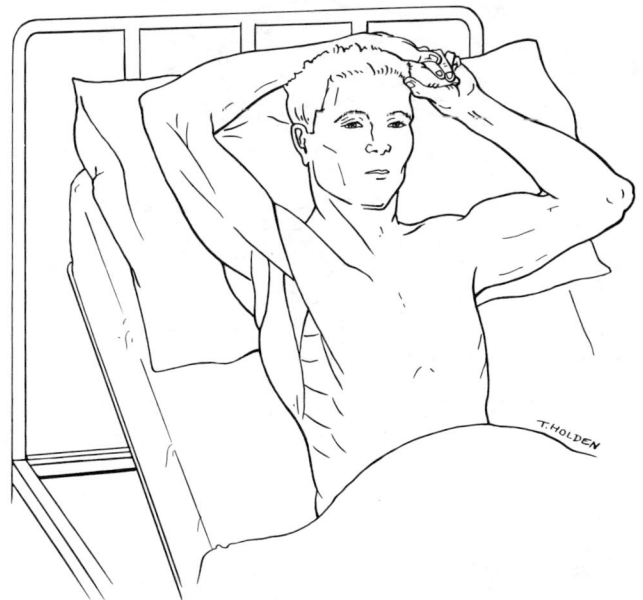

Figure 3.1.

Patient position for right-sided lateral thoracentesis. Correct interspace in midaxillary line is selected by percussion of fluid level.

fourth intercostal space, midclavicular line, and very rarely on the left side, because of the heart. To locate the interspace, first palpate the sternal protuberance where the second rib meets the sternum—the angle of Louis. The interspace directly inferior to the second rib is the second interspace.

Another satisfactory approach is the posterior one (Figure 3.2). The patient is seated on the edge of the bed, leaning forward (to pull the scapulae anteriorly), with his head and arms comfortably supported by a pillow on an adjustable stand. The physician stands on the opposite side of the bed and makes his puncture about 2.5 inches lateral to the spinous processes, below the tip of the scapula. At this point, the paraspinal musculature will prevent accurate delineation of intercostal spaces. Percuss both lung fields to

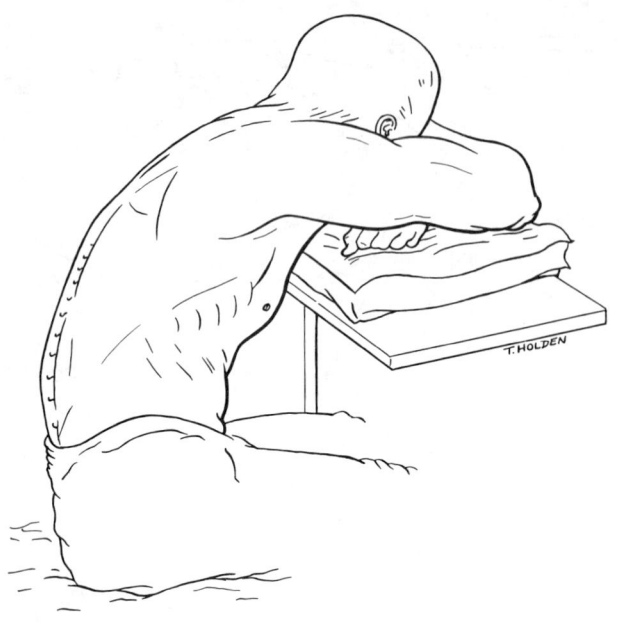

Figure 3.2.

Patient position for posterior thoracentesis. Puncture should be lateral to vertical bulk of paraspinal musculature.

determine the level of dullness of the affected side, *and then pass the needle through one interspace higher than this level.* The most common mistake made in this procedure is to go too low, and this method of determining the proper interspace is applicable wherever on the chest the puncture is made. Pleural fluid rises in a meniscus where it touches parietal pleura; this is often visible on the chest x-ray. Penetration at the level of this meniscus will allow full drainage with less danger of diaphragmatic penetration or of being in the diaphragmatic sulcus and sealed off from the fluid by lung tissue above the needle. As the lung expands, it will tend to push the fluid along the meniscus curve upward to the needle tip.

Hands should be washed and sterile gloves worn. A wide area of the skin is cleansed, in the event that more than one pass is required, and towels are used as drapes, with one on the bed serving as an instrument table. The thoracentesis flask should be sitting close by on the bed, or preferably, held at the ready by an assistant. A wheal of local anesthetic is raised with the 25-gauge needle at the proposed puncture site, and the 20-gauge needle is then used for deeper infiltration. Even in the muscular or obese individual, the 1.5-inch length of this needle will usually reach and penetrate the pleura. It should be advanced perpendicular to the skin, with constant infiltration, until it strikes the rib forming the lower border of the selected interspace. The point is now redirected to pass *immediately above* the bone, thereby avoiding the intercostal bundle of vessels and nerve that run along the inferior surface of each rib. The pleura is sensitive, and should be carefully anesthetized. As the physician passes through it, a slight "give" can usually be felt, and, if correctly located, pleural fluid may be aspirated.

Remove the needle. Attach the three-way stopcock to the 50-ml syringe and secure the 15-gauge or 17-gauge needle to the stopcock. Use the larger bore if the initial return was purulent or fibrinous. Test the stopcock; its use allows the physician to perform the thoracentesis without exposing the pleural cavity to the air. After attaching the 18-gauge needle to the rubber tubing on the side arm, the long 15-gauge or 17-gauge needle is advanced along the anesthetized tract until pleural fluid is aspirated. A nick in the skin with the no. 11 blade may facilitate passage through the skin.

There is no reason to advance the needle tip more than a few millimeters into the pleural cavity. In fact, if the fluid meniscus has been picked up, further penetration will usually only impale the lung. To prevent inadvertent advancement, clamp the needle with the Kelly clamp flush against the skin (Figure 3.3). The first samples drawn are used for bacterial cultures.

If the thoracentesis is for diagnostic purposes only, the three-way stopcock is not required. A sterile 10-ml syringe containing 200 units of sterile heparin is attached directly to the thoracentesis needle before the pleura is penetrated. After the pleural cavity is entered, the syringe is filled, and

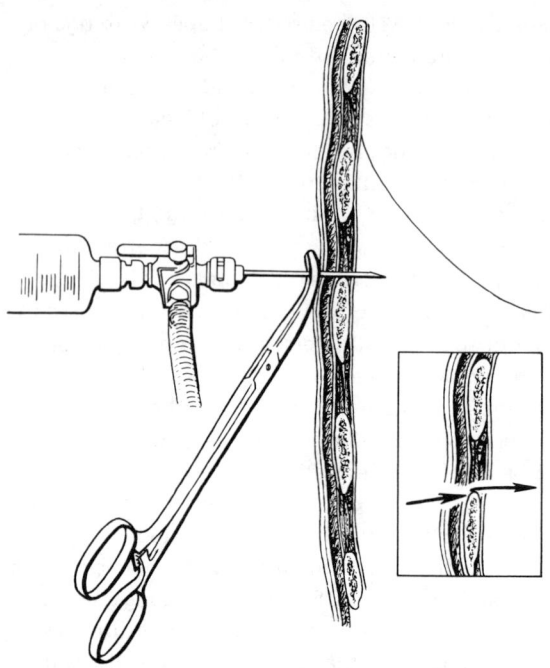

Figure 3.3.

Thoracentesis. Clamp prevents overpenetration by needle. Inset: Needle path impinges upon, then passes above rib to avoid intercostal neurovascular bundle.

the needle is withdrawn, removed from the syringe, and replaced with a shorter needle with a sterile protective cover. The syringe is taken immediately to the laboratory for examination of cells and bacteria, and for indicated cultures.

If the evacuated thoracentesis flask is fitted with a nipple, the 18-gauge needle on the rubber tubing may be thrust through it, and the stopcock turned to allow the fluid to be sucked directly into the bottle. Often the fastest way is repeatedly to fill the syringe and then expel the fluid through the side arm into the opened flask.

As the fluid is exhausted, the visceral pleura will begin to strike the needle tip with a palpable, and frequently audible, fluttering. The appearance of some bubbles of air shortly thereafter in the syringe means that the needle is in peripheral lung tissue, but not that a significant pneumothorax is in the offing. Most leaks of this type seal spontaneously, but these two signs are clear indications to change the needle position. Coughing, common at this stage, will also tend to impale the lung; warn the patient to resist the impulse. Surprisingly, redirecting the angle of the needle, withdrawing it a few millimeters, or simply rotating the syringe to change the direction of the open bevel will often yield several hundred more milliliters of drainage, and these maneuvers should always be tried before final removal.

If the yield clearly is less than that estimated as present, repeat the tap in the next lower interspace, or in a different position. Do not exhaust the patient, however, with prolonged and repeated attempts; rarely is thoracentesis such an emergency that it cannot be tried again later. If anticancer medications are to be instilled into the pleural cavity, some fluid is necessary to ensure even distribution of the drug. In these cases, do not remove all possible fluid first, and instruct the patient to change positions frequently after instillation. A simple Band-Aid is the only dressing required. The fluid is sent for appropriate cytologic and biochemical studies (see Collection of Cytology Specimens, Section 4.5).

The most common hazard associated with thoracentesis is a pneumothorax. Steps to avoid this were discussed under Technique, but it is accurate to say that even the most scrupulous doctor will cause this complication, often a reflection of the disease process itself, if he does enough thoracenteses. Because the air leak may not be clinically obvious (or clinically significant), a chest film shortly after every tap is a wise precaution, alerting the physician to the presence of air and the percentage of lung collapse, as well as the percentage of fluid removed.

Other less frequent complications include:

Intrathoracic Bleeding
This condition is most often due to parenchymal pulmonary injury, but occasionally to a damaged intercostal artery.

Careful placement of the thoracentesis needle will avoid the latter, and bloody return via the needle after an initially serous drainage usually indicates that the needle tip is now penetrating lung tissue and should be withdrawn. Bleeding in the patient on the short-acting anticoagulant, heparin, can be minimized by timing the thoracentesis to occur just prior to the next scheduled dose, i.e., when the clotting time is least prolonged.

Visceral Injuries
Damage to the liver, spleen, and other intra-abdominal organs can occur when the needle is passed through too low an interspace and penetrates the diaphragm, or when the diaphragm is abnormally elevated. Although the interspace selected depends upon the location of the fluid, it is rarely necessary to go lower than the sixth in the standard mid-axillary approach. Diseases which cause splenic or hepatic enlargement should lead to special care in interspace selection. The aspiration of blood that clots should alert the physician to the possibility of liver or spleen injury.

Pleural Contamination
The inadvertent spread of infection into the pleural cavity by aspiration of a pulmonary or subphrenic abscess is a rare complication if the patient's clinical course, physical findings, and x-ray examinations are adequately reviewed prior to drainage. Its potentially disastrous consequences, however, are further proofs of the importance of accurate fluid localization before the tap.

Protein Depletion
It should be remembered that the protein content of serous pleural effusions, particularly malignant ones, is relatively high. Repeated "therapeutic" taps can rapidly exhaust the cancer patient's already enfeebled reserve. If the effusion fails to respond to medical therapy and is not the cause of respiratory embarrassment, it is better in such cases not to "tap it dry."

Pleural Shock

Although patients may become hypotensive and faint for a variety of reasons during thoracentesis, true pleural shock is an extremely rare complication. Presumably it is caused by the needle penetrating a pulmonary vein, producing a fistula, with air embolus. Treatment is supportive, with the patient kept head down and on his right side in an effort to trap the bubbles in the left ventricle.

3.2. THORACOSTOMY

The position and type of chest tube used for a thoracostomy will be dictated by the clinical condition treated. Even though a pneumothorax requires a different approach than a hemothorax, the principle applying to both is that the tube be equal to the task. When intrathoracic bleeding or pus is diagnosed, the insertion of a catheter smaller than a no. 20 French will prove inadequate. For a hydrothorax requiring tube drainage, a no. 16 French tube is usually sufficient, and a no. 14 French tube will handle most cases of pneumothorax.

MATERIAL

A sterilized thoracostomy kit containing nos. 1 and 2 trocars of the Nelson type (a no. 1 will accept a no. 14 French and a no. 2 will accept a no. 20 French catheter), forceps, Kelly clamp, nos. 14, 16, and 20 French 16-inch red rubber or Bardic catheters (the latter are stiffer and will resist collapse if suction is to be used), ampules of local anesthetic, 10-ml syringe, 25-gauge and 22-gauge needles, scalpel handle, no. 11 blade, skin stitches, scissors, towels, connectors to fit the catheters to drainage tubing, sterile gauze pads. Floor supplies: sterile drainage tubing, underwater-seal bottle, sterile gloves, antiseptic solution, tape.

Comment. The Argyle plastic thoracostomy tube with enclosed trocar is an excellent unit and eliminates the need for separate trocars and catheters.

TECHNIQUE
*Hemothorax, Hydrothorax,
or Empyema*

Although loculated fluid will occasionally require unusual positioning of the tube, most cases are best drained with the patient in the position for a lateral thoracentesis (see Figure 3.1), supine if in shock, and with the tube entering the chest in the midaxillary line at the sixth intercostal space. X-rays are an important guide and should be obtained first whenever feasible. The site chosen should be far enough anterior so that the patient will be able to lie comfortably on his back without kinking the tube.

Sterile gloves and mask are worn, and the lateral thorax is widely prepared. An assistant is useful, though not essential. A wheal of anesthesia is raised, and the infiltration is carried deeper with the 22-gauge needle, impinging upon the rib and then passing immediately above it to avoid the intercostal bundle of vessels and nerves. Aspirate as the needle penetrates the pleura to confirm proper placement, and anesthetize the pleura thoroughly.

Prepare the no. 20 or no. 16 French catheter by cutting several additional side holes over the first 4 inches. If a Bardic or similar plastic catheter is chosen, the stiff, flaring end must have an ellipse removed to allow it to pass through the sleeve of the trocar (Figure 3.4A), and it should be tested for ease of passage before inserting the trocar. Measure the length of catheter that must be advanced before the the last side hole passes the inner end of the trocar, and clamp the other end of the tube in the shank of the Kelly clamp at a point that will allow this length to protrude.

Nick the skin with the scalpel and place a skin stitch, as illustrated in Figure 3.5, before passing the trocar. Introduce the no. 2 Nelson or similar trocar at right angles to the skin through this short incision, again impinging upon, then passing over, the rib (Figure 3.4B). A light rotary motion will ease the passage, and a definite "give" will be palpable as the pleura is penetrated; do not advance suddenly as this happens. Remove the trocar, advance the sleeve about one centimeter, and observe the initial efflux, obtaining cultures

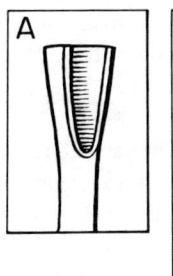
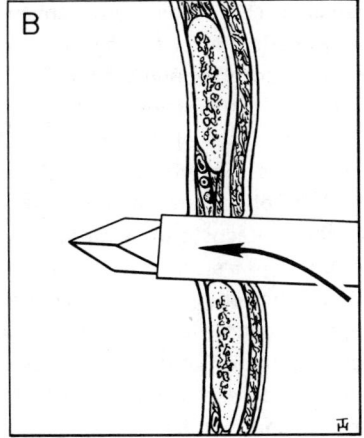

Figure 3.4.

(**A**) Ellipse cut in flaring end of catheter, necessary when stiff plastic catheters are used. (**B**) Passage of Nelson trocar. Note that tip passes immediately above the superior border of the rib to avoid injury to the intercostal neurovascular bundle.

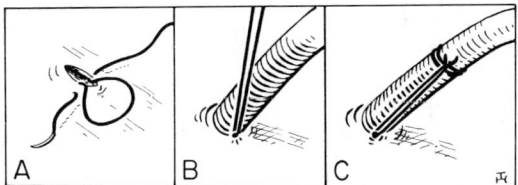

Figure 3.5.

Securing stitch for intercostal tube. (**A**) Stitch is placed prior to passage of catheter. (**B**) After tube is in place, stitch is tied first to snug incision, then (**C**) is tied about catheter to prevent slippage. When the catheter is removed, only the second tie is cut.

at this time if desired. Insert the chest tube through the sleeve the full distance to the Kelly clamp. Remove the Kelly clamp, begin to pull out the metal sleeve, and immediately shift the clamp to the tubing showing between the sleeve and the skin, holding it there while the sleeve is further removed to prevent inadvertent removal of the catheter as well. Advance the chest tube about 2 cm and immediately tie down the skin stitch after testing for adequate flow. This single stitch serves both to snug the incision around the tube and to anchor it in position.

During the performance of this procedure, the assistant should have prepared the underwater-seal bottle to receive the catheter. If the physician is alone, he should prepare the bottle before the thoracostomy, wrapping the open end of the drainage tubing in a sterile towel to prevent contamination. The further the tubing is submerged beneath the water in the bottle, the greater the pressure must be in the pleural space to allow evacuation of its contents. The end should be only 2 cm below the surface (Figure 3.6), and the whole apparatus, in free communication with the pleural space, must be maintained as a sterile unit. Should a pleural suc-

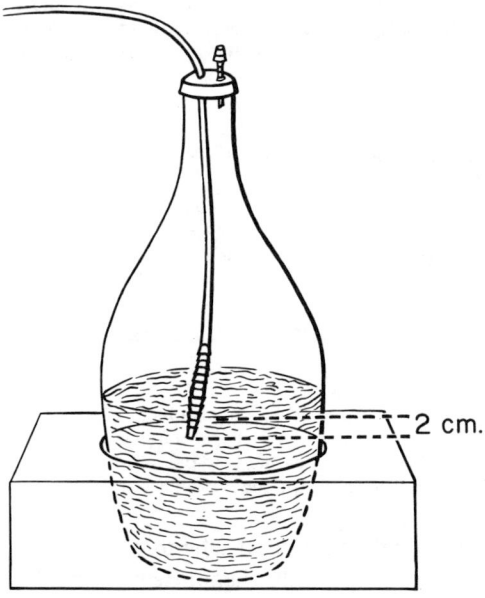

Figure 3.6.

Underwater-seal drainage. Catheter tip should remain approximately 2 cm beneath fluid surface, and bottle should be fitted in a case or firmly taped to the floor to prevent tipping with loss of seal.

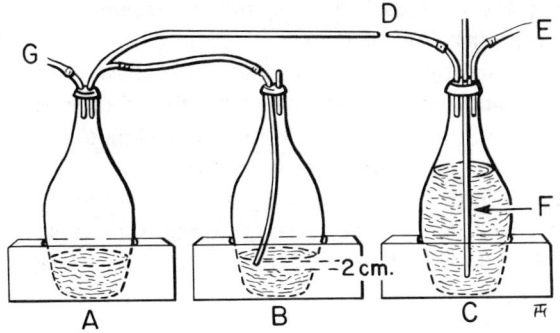

Figure 3.7.

Three-bottle system for underwater seal and suction. Bottle **A** traps and holds fluid drained. Bottle **B** is the underwater seal. Suction is regulated by the depth of tube **F** beneath the surface of the fluid in bottle **C**. Tube **E** is connected to suction source or clamped at **D** if only underwater seal is used. Tube **G** is connected to the intercostal catheter.

tion pump, such as the Emerson unit, not be available, the use of the 3-bottle drainage system (Figure 3.7) allows the later use of simple wall suction if required. However, the cumbersome nature of the three-bottle system has led to its widespread replacement by portable units now made of extruded plastic, such as that illustrated in Figure 3.8, the Pleur-evac, manufactured by the Krale division of Deknatel. The physiologic principles of these convenient units remain the same. Fit a connector piece, if necessary, to both the catheter and drainage tubing, *tape both junctions well,* remove the clamp, and apply a light dressing with additional split lengths of tape to fix the tube in place.

A no. 16 or no. 14 French catheter in this position may also be used to advantage in the treatment by drugs of malignant effusions. After the drainage of the bulk, but not all, of the effusion, the selected drug is instilled via the chest tube into the pleural cavity, the tube clamped, and the patient turned frequently over the next 24-hour period to assure its even distribution. At the conclusion, the remaining fluid is drained, allowing the treated pleural surfaces to become coapted. The catheter is then removed. Although the same goal can be reached by separate thoracenteses, drainage is probably less adequate.

Note. Crush injuries or bullet wounds of the chest, with massive bleeding, may require larger tubes than those possible via the sleeve of the Nelson trocar. Such catheters may be easily introduced between the spread jaws of a Kelly clamp, thrust into the pleural space in the same manner as the trocar. Both fluid and air losses can occur in these cases, and therefore both posterior and anterior chest tubes may be needed.

Pneumothorax

It is beyond the purpose of this manual to discuss the indications for the use of a chest tube in cases of pneumothorax. The issue is not a settled one. Many cases require no treatment, some may be adequately handled by simple aspiration, and a tension pneumothorax requires tube drainage. Beyond these rather unhelpful generalities, however, will be the specifics of the individual case. Past history and clinical severity, whatever the type of pneumothorax, will help to dictate the proper course. Remember that tube drainage in reality is the most conservative treatment, and it is the safest course in borderline cases.

Once the decision for catheterization has been reached, a no. 14 French red rubber or Bardic-type catheter is preferable to an Intracath. Many cases of pneumothorax will eventually be associated with a pleural effusion that can plug small catheters, and the flexibility of the Intracath makes it difficult to direct with any accuracy.

The general technique is precisely the same as described above, but the location of the tube is different, and the patient is in a semisitting position. Because intrapleural air will rise unless trapped, the tip of the catheter should lie over the apex of the lung. The most direct approach to this area is via the second intercostal space (opposite the sternal angle of Louis), in the midclavicular line. The no. 1 trocar is used, and again several extra holes are cut in the first four inches of the catheter. An additional and useful safeguard is to place a silk tie around the tube at a distance from the most proximal hole somewhat greater than the estimated thickness of the chest wall. This guide will ensure that the tube is advanced until the final side hole is intrapleural and not subcutaneous. The latter position, particularly in the presence of a tension pneumothorax, can lead to the rapid and dramatic appearance of subcutaneous emphysema. The preplaced skin stitch, when tied, will also help to prevent this.

The patient is first placed on simple underwater-seal drainage (see Figure 3.6), and if the lung subsequently fails to reexpand adequately, negative pressure may be applied via the Emerson pump, 3-bottle suction (see Figure 3.7), or a Pleur-evac type unit (see Figure 3.8). If longer than 48 hours of drainage is required, prophylactic antibiotics are started.

An acceptable alternate incision, particularly in women, is in the third intercostal space, just lateral and well posterior to the pectoralis major muscle (Figure 3.9). By starting somewhat lower than the midclavicular approach, it actually affords a better uphill guide toward the thoracic apex, and it leaves a considerably less conspicuous scar.

Intermittent milking or irrigation of the chest tube may be required to assure continuous function, particularly for a hemothorax or after chest surgery. The latter should be done only by a physician, maintaining sterile technique. Chest tubes should be clamped when the patient is being moved, but never for a prolonged period in cases of pneumothorax or bronchopleural fistula, as this can result in a tension pneumothorax. Such patients, therefore, should have portable x-ray studies. To prevent syphoning of fluid from the bottle into the patient, never lift the bottle above the level of the patient's chest unless the tubing is clamped. Always use an atraumatic chest tube clamp or the shank (not jaws) of a Kelly clamp. As the fluid level rises in a single underwater-seal bottle, the tubing should be carefully withdrawn to maintain its tip approximately 2 cm below the surface. When opacity of the pleural drainage prevents direct visualization, the use of a plastic connector, fitted into the submerged end, will alert the physician when the

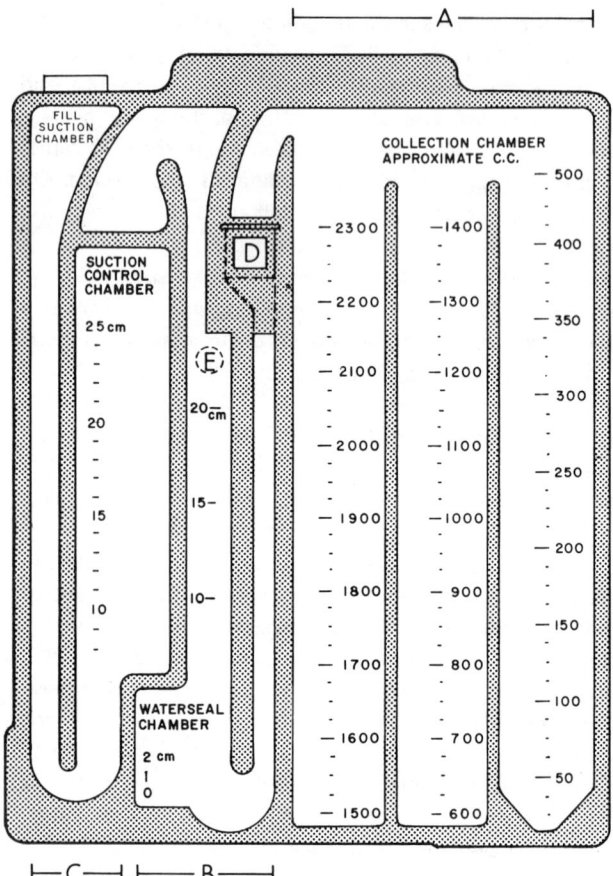

Figure 3.8.

A typical plastic portable underwater-seal drainage unit. The right-hand portion **A** contains the pleural drainage; the center section **B** contains the underwater seal. Suction tubing may be connected directly to the unit, and the degree of suction is controlled by the water level in section **C**. In this unit, a float valve at **D** prevents the patient from breaking the underwater seal by exerting excessive negative intrapleural pressure. A small positive-pressure release valve at **E** is closed under suction but opens under positive pressure to eliminate the possibility of tension pneumothorax in the case of blocked suction, and to prevent water loss in the suction chamber when the patient coughs.

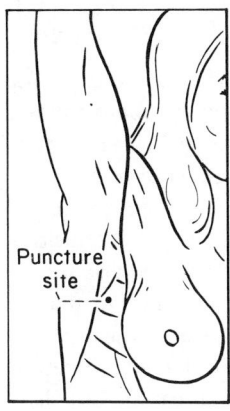

Figure 3.9.

Axillary approach for high intercostal catheter. The third or fourth interspace is selected. Note that puncture site is well posterior to the pectoralis major muscle.

tip nears the surface. If underwater-seal bottles are used, they should be fitted firmly in a case (see Figures 3.6, 3.7) to prevent inadvertent overturning and loss of seal.

Removal of Chest Tubes

Chest tubes should be removed when they no longer function. Turn the patient so that the tube is superior to the lung (semisitting for anterior tubes, lateral decubitus for midaxillary tubes). Have several pretorn strips of adhesive within reach, and prepare a double-layered dressing of an inner alcohol-moistened sponge and an outer layer of dry gauze. Petroleum-jelly-impregnated dressings are not necessary.

Cut the stitch about the catheter, but leave the portion coapting the skin edges. Now ask the patient to take a deep breath and hold it. This Valsalva maneuver will prevent aspiration of air as the tube is removed. Rapidly withdraw the catheter while the patient is holding his breath, and immediately place the dressing over the exit site and tape it in place.

3.3. PERICARDIAL PUNCTURE

A pericardial puncture may be a diagnostic tool in the work-up of an obscure pericardial effusion, or, in the treatment of acute cardiac tamponade, life-saving therapy. This potentially lethal complication of injury or disease requires swift relief once the classic signs of tamponade are recognized. Although the disorders associated with pericardial effusions are the most common causes, tamponade should also be suspected in all patients with penetrating wounds of the chest. Radiologic examination is a vital asset in the evaluation of pericardial effusions, not only for the determination of cardiac silhouette and presence of calcification, but also for the fluoroscopic observation of the cardiac excursions, markedly reduced in the presence of either excessive pericardial fluid or constrictive pericarditis.

Whenever possible, the patient should be followed throughout the procedure with an electrocardiograph. The appearance of an "injury potential" or ventricular premature contractions on the tracing, as the needle contacts the epicardium, gives the physician warning to withdraw the tip until these changes disappear. The ST segment elevation is seen most clearly on the electrocardiograph when the V setting is used, and the chest lead is directly connected to the needle, which then functions as an electrode probe. A conducting wire with alligator clamps on either end, kept available in a sterilized pack, is useful for this procedure. In addition, when performing a pericardial tap in cases for which the distinction between thickened pericardium and pericardial effusion is in doubt, the safety of fluoroscopic monitoring is useful.

MATERIAL
Four-inch short-beveled 18-gauge needle, 50-ml syringe, local anesthetic and syringe for skin infiltration, sterile container for aspirate, antiseptic-soaked sponges, gloves.
Comment. Once the pericardium is penetrated, a catheter may be inserted through the needle for aspiration, and the needle withdrawn. Although theoretically safer, it requires

the use of a 16-gauge needle to allow passage of a PE 160 or 190 catheter. A large-bore Intracath or Rochester-type needle may also be used.

TECHNIQUE

The patient is in bed with his head elevated 30 to 40 degrees to assist drainage. A nurse should be in attendance, and the electrocardiograph in clear view, or preferably watched by an assistant. Gloves should be worn.

An area immediately to the left of the xyphoid process and inferior to the lowest rib is cleansed and infiltrated with local anesthetic. The aspirating needle is now introduced at an angle of 20 degrees to the skin, which will carry the tip just beneath the sternum, and is advanced at this depth along an imaginary line between the point of entry and the patient's *right* shoulder. A tough, elastic resistance will be felt as the needle penetrates the diaphragm, and thereafter progress should be cautious, with frequent aspirations and close observation of the electrocardiograph. If the pericardium is not badly thickened, cardiac pulsations are often palpably transmitted via the needle as it impinges on the pericardial surface.

The nature of the initial return is noted. It may be impossible to distinguish a bloody pericardial effusion from inadvertent puncture of the right ventricle. Before the needle is removed, such fluid should be sent for immediate determination of its hematocrit, with the expectation of a low hematocrit from an effusion. Bloody pericardial fluid may clot, but if some fluid is placed in a test tube and does not clot, the needle is not penetrating the ventricles. An initially clear return will often become blood-tinged as it is drawn off, indicating some mild degree of fresh bleeding secondary to the procedure, and is not a cause for alarm.

After removal only of as much fluid as needed without undue manipulation of the tip, *and with certainty of proper needle position,* 50 cc of air may be injected into the pericardial sac to aid in x-ray studies of the heart. The needle is removed, the fluid is sent for appropriate studies, and the patient is kept under close observation for signs of recurring tamponade. Disease states that require two pericardial taps within 24 hours, or in which the fluid is too thick or fibrinous for adequate aspiration, will almost invariably require pericardiotomy.

Aspiration of the pericardial sac may also be performed through the left fourth intercostal space, the needle passing at right angles to the chest wall at a point 4 cm lateral to the sternal border. It has three potential disadvantages: (1) the internal mammary artery may be abnormally placed or may be branching at this level, and can be injured; (2) the pleura may be entered (without consequence, unless air is allowed to leak in during the procedure, or unless a fistula is thereby established between the pleural space and a purulent pericardial effusion); and (3) the left anterior descending coronary artery can be injured.

3.4. ABDOMINAL PARACENTESIS

Diagnostic Abdominal Taps

Although of little usefulness in mechanical obstruction or localized abscesses, diagnostic abdominal taps are clearly indicated in cases of suspected intra-abdominal hemorrhage or generalized peritonitis of unknown etiology. Should the clinical examination or x-rays suggest diffuse and massive bowel dilatation, an abdominal tap is hazardous and likely to yield only intestinal gas. Similarly, patients with known or likely widespread adhesions make poor candidates for abdominal taps, and areas of previous incisions should be avoided as likely to mask locally adherent loops.

The abdomen should first be carefully examined for fluid localization and for the presence of abnormally enlarged organs, in order to avoid inadvertent biopsies and to fix in the mind of the physician the limits of the peritoneal reflections. Paracentesis sites should be lateral to the vertical borders of the rectus muscle. As a general guide only, Figure 3.10 illustrates acceptable positions for four-quadrant taps.

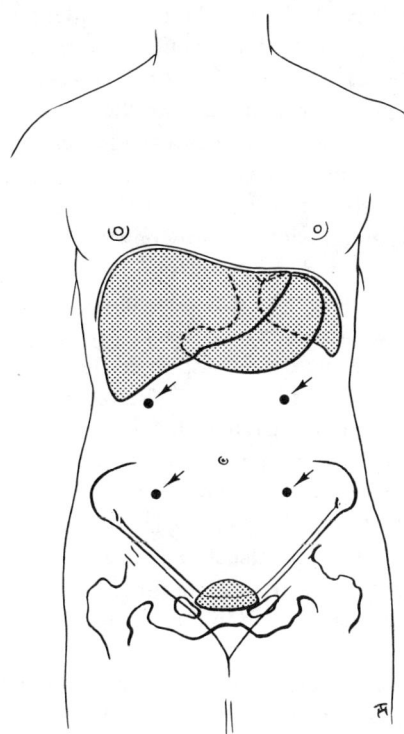

Figure 3.10.

Sites for four-quadrant abdominal taps. Abnormally enlarged organs will alter these locations. To avoid injury to the epigastric vessels, puncture sites are lateral to the lateral borders of the rectus muscle.

MATERIAL

Sterile 18-gauge spinal needle with obturator, syringe, local anesthetic in separate syringe with 25-gauge needle, culture tubes, microscope slides, and antiseptic solution.

TECHNIQUE

Immediately after voiding, the patient is placed in the supine position. If the physician is not satisfied by clinical examination that the bladder is decompressed, it should be catheterized before proceeding.

The entire abdomen is now cleansed, and local anesthesia infiltrated to, and including, the peritoneum in each quadrant at the four selected sites. With the obturator in place, the spinal needle is now passed at right angles to the skin in the quadrant the physician's clinical judgment assesses as most likely to yield information. A firm resistance, then "give," will be clearly palpable as the peritoneum is penetrated; be prepared for it and do not suddenly pass too deep. Remove the obturator, and watch for spontaneous efflux. If there is none, gentle suction may be applied to the needle, but there is little to be gained by advancing the tip. Each quadrant is aspirated in succession. Aspirated fluid should be checked for blood and submitted for suitable bacteriologic and chemical studies. Gram stains should be performed by the physician. Occasionally, small fluid collections may be picked up by turning the patient on his side, allowing the fluid to drain, and then tapping the lower side while the patient remains in the decubitus position (e.g., patients with suspected liver trauma are turned with the left side down, and are then tapped in the left upper or lower quadrants).

Should an obvious bowel perforation be produced, simply remove the needle; it is a comforting thought that the great majority of such injuries seal rapidly, even in the presence of mechanical obstruction, and require only close observation for 24 hours. Negative taps by no means rule out the presence of significant bleeding; if negative results do not support the clinical impression, the doctor should act on the assumption that bleeding is present.

A more recent variation of this technique, designed to increase the diagnostic yield and minimize potential hazard to the patient, is the use of the peritoneal dialysis catheter for diagnostic peritoneal lavage. As in the technique already described, previous surgical procedures are a relative contraindication; and the bladder must be emptied, in the unconscious or uncooperative patient, by catheterization.

The abdomen is prepared as for therapeutic paracentesis, described below. Under local anesthesia, a skin incision is made in the midline, midway between the umbilicus and the symphysis pubis. The dialysis catheter, with trocar inserted, is then introduced in the midline through this incision, using a twisting motion of the trocar, until the tip is felt to penetrate the plastic resistance of the peritoneum. Depth of penetration should be controlled by grasping the catheter with the thumb and index finger. The stylet is removed and the curved distal tip of the catheter is advanced into the right or left pelvic gutter. For greater rigidity, the stylet may be only partially withdrawn (to 1 1/2 inches) while placing the catheter. The connecting tubing is now attached, and one liter of saline solution is introduced into the abdomen. Turn the patient from side to side. The tubing is then lowered over the side of the bed after an equilibration time of 5 minutes. The color of the fluid is noted as it is returned and the presence of bleeding, free bile, or feces confirmed.

The theoretical advantage of this procedure is that localized bleeding areas, unreached by four-quadrant taps, may be detected by the wider distribution of the fluid used in this technique. Like any diagnostic test, this procedure should be used to confirm clinical findings. Blind adherence to the results of this test will lead, on occasion, to unnecessary surgery. Although there is little doubt that the return of dark, wine-colored fluid indicates the presence of significant abdominal bleeding, it is not unusual for the fluid to return with a slightly pink cast, suggesting some intra-abdominal hemorrhage. The significance of such hemorrhage may be minimal; it should not be an indication for immediate surgery unless physical signs suggesting major intra-abdominal hemorrhage are present. The presence of intra-abdominal bleeding is quite common in trauma, and in the absence of deteriorating or localizing abdominal findings it should indicate the need for careful, repeated observation rather than for rapid exploration.

Therapeutic Paracentesis

The availability of increasingly effective oral diuretics and antitumor drugs, and the recognition of the hazard of protein depletion, have led to a decline in the indications for the use of therapeutic paracentesis in the treatment of cirrhotic and malignant ascites. Intractable, symptomatic ascites is not, however, a vanished affliction, and the judicial use of the trocar in the proper patient can afford considerable relief.

MATERIAL

Sterilized paracentesis kit containing Dukes trocar with connected tubing (Figure 3.11), 5-ml syringe, 25-gauge and 22-gauge needles, towels, sponges, ampules of local anesthetic, scalpel handle, no. 11 blade, and 4-0 silk skin stitches. Floor supplies: skin disinfectant, sterile gloves, large basin, and barrier drapes.

TECHNIQUE

The patient usually is sitting on the edge of his bed with legs dangling. The bladder must first be emptied. If necessary, the lower half of the abdomen should be shaved before cleansing the skin. Prepare a wide area that includes both lower quadrants, and cover both legs with the barrier drapes. Gloves should be worn.

Infiltrate local anesthesia down to the peritoneum at a point in the midline, halfway between the symphysis pubis and the umbilicus, and then make a small nick in the skin here to facilitate the passage of the trocar. The metal sleeve with trocar in place is now passed through this opening at a right angle to the skin. A tough resistance, then "give," will

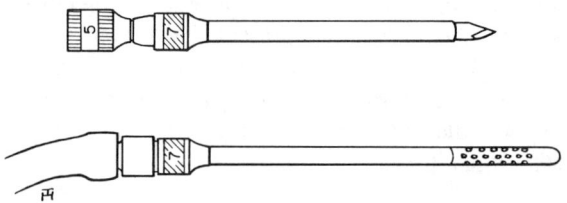

Figure 3.11.

Dukes trocar. Fenestrated sleeve prevents clogging by entrapped omentum.

usually be felt as the peritoneum is penetrated. Once this is passed, remove the obturator and fit in the fenestrated inner sleeve; this allows free passage of fluid without permitting omentum to clog the open tip. The rubber tubing is led to the basin, and the fluid is allowed to flow freely. The patient's vital signs should be monitored during paracentesis. Massive ascites, which should not be totally drained at one sitting, should be eliminated with intermittent periods of clamping of the tube to prevent the shocklike state occasionally produced if the fluid shifts are too rapid. At the conclusion, bending the patient from side to side may produce additional fluid from the lateral peritoneal gutters.

On removal of the trocar, the incision may require a stitch to prevent excessive leakage of residual peritoneal fluid, and it is not unusual for some fluid to escape for several days. The specimen may be sent for appropriate cytologic examination in the case of suspected but unproved malignant ascites (see Collection of Cytology Specimens, Section 4.5). Apply an absorbent dressing.

Note. When it appears that frequently repeated paracenteses will be necessary, a large-bore Intracath may be used in place of the Dukes trocar, and the catheter taped in place after removal of the needle, for future use. An antibiotic jelly is applied at the site of entrance, and a dry dressing taped in place.

3.5. CULDOCENTESIS

Aspiration of the pouch of Douglas through the posterior fornix is a valuable procedure in the diagnosis of ectopic pregnancy. Although the absence of blood does not eliminate the possible existence of tubal pregnancy, its presence is presumptive evidence for the diagnosis, warranting laparotomy.

MATERIAL
Vaginal speculum, tenaculum, 18-gauge lumbar puncture needle, 10-ml syringe, gloves, lubricant.

TECHNIQUE

A sedative may be given beforehand, but it is not required. The patient is placed in lithotomy position on a gynecologic examining table, and the operator is seated comfortably at the end of the table. Although culdocentesis may be accomplished in bed, using an overturned bedpan beneath the buttocks to elevate the perineum, this technique is definitely less satisfactory. Lighting, either by gooseneck lamp or flashlight, must be adequate.

A careful bimanual pelvic examination precedes culdocentesis. Frequently, blood in the cul de sac causes a doughy fullness that is easily palpable in the posterior fornix.

After insertion of the vaginal speculum, the posterior lip of the cervix is grasped with the tenaculum and is gently swept anteriorly. The proper site for needle puncture is midline in the posterior fornix, just where the vaginal mucosa meets the cervix. This fold may be made more obvious by carefully pushing the cervix in and out with the tenaculum. The needle, attached to the syringe, is inserted at this point, and directed posteriorly, usually on an angle of about 45 degrees to the patient's frontal plane. A slight "give" will often be felt as the peritoneum is punctured. Aspirated fluid is then examined grossly for blood.

Early resistance and inability to obtain fluid usually indicate that the needle is burrowing into the cervix or uterus, and needs to be redirected more posteriorly. Extreme degrees of retroversion, or obliteration of the cul de sac by previous inflammation or endometriosis, may make aspiration difficult or impossible. The pelvic examination will forewarn the operator of the presence of either of these conditions.

3.6. JOINT ASPIRATION AND SYNOVIAL BIOPSY

The indications for entering a joint space with a needle are both diagnostic and therapeutic. Aspiration can produce valuable information about the etiology of many joint effusions. Although the fluid itself yields the most important knowledge, synovial biopsies can also aid in the diagnosis of properly selected cases, *if the pathology department is experienced in interpreting them.* Few cases of rheumatoid arthritis require this technique to establish the diagnosis; it is of greatest use in the identification of tuberculosis, sarcoidosis, fungal arthritides, hemosiderosis, and certain orthopedic conditions, the most important of which is villonodular synovitis. The injection of a contrast medium (usually 50 percent Renografin) and air for arthogram studies of the knee and other joints can be useful in the diagnosis of obscure injuries, *if the radiology department is experienced in interpreting them.*

Aspirations are therapeutically effective in the relief of pain from acute joint distension, secondary either to trauma or infection, and the intra-articular injection of steroids is indicated in the treatment of certain joint conditions. Although the use of local antibiotics in the therapy of septic arthritis continues, its theoretical basis is somewhat vague. It has been demonstrated that systematically administered antibiotics enter the inflamed joint space in adequate concentrations; septic effusions that do not respond rapidly to such treatment usually require surgical incision and drainage. Local skin and soft tissue infections or bacteremia are contraindications to this technique.

MATERIAL

Four-inch 22-gauge needle (for joint injection and infiltration of anesthetic), 4-inch 18-gauge needle (for joint aspiration), 10-ml Luer-Lok syringe, ampules of local anesthetic, sterile gloves, antiseptic-soaked sponges, 10 percent formalin in biopsy jars, filter paper, culture tubes, slides, test tubes.

TECHNIQUE

The occasional incidence of joint infection, particularly following the use of hydrocortisone, reflects failure to maintain strict aseptic technique. Gloves must be worn, and skin preparation must be thorough. *Infiltration of local anesthesia should include the pain-sensitive joint capsule.*

Knee

The swollen knee joint may be approached from either its medial or lateral side, although the latter is safer, avoiding possible injury to the saphenous nerve. With the knee fully extended, the needle is introduced into the suprapatellar bursa approximately 2 cm above the lateral superior border of the patella, parallel with the skin surface and passing deep to the bone. Pressure exerted by the free hand on the opposite (medial) side of the joint can make the synovium bulge more prominently.

Hip

Two approaches are acceptable. The puncture site for the anterior approach is 2 cm below the inguinal ligament, a thumb width lateral to the femoral pulse. The patient lies supine, with his patella straight up, and the needle passes through the anesthetized wheal at right angles to the skin. For the lateral approach the needle travels a slightly cephalad course parallel with the femoral neck, from a point 1.5 cm below the greater trochanter, anterior to the ischial tuberosity, and in a plane parallel with the table. The point should pass through the adductors and close to the neck of the femur.

Elbow

Because of its limited distensibility, fluid in the elbow joint rapidly becomes apparent as a lateral swelling. The puncture site is a point equidistant from the olecranon, lateral epicondyle, and radial head. The elbow is flexed at a right angle prior to aspiration.

Shoulder

This joint is approached from its anterior aspect, at a spot approximately a fingerbreadth lateral to the coracoid process. The needle penetrates the skin at right angles.

Wrist

The radiocarpal compartment of this joint may be entered from the dorsal aspect of the wrist by passing a needle at right angles to the skin, immediately distal to the head of the radius, and between the two tendons of the extensor pollicis longus and extensor indicis proprius.

Ankle

The ankle joint can be approached from either the anteromedial aspect (between the medial border of the tibialis anterior and the medial malleolus), or the anterolateral aspect (between the lateral border of the peronaeus tertius and the lateral malleolus). In both instances the needle is passed on a gentle decline to gain access to the joint between the tibia and the talus.

Note. The appearance of fluid is the best indication that the joint has been entered. If no fluid is forthcoming, and the anatomic position appears correct, a small amount of sterile saline solution may be injected and aspirated.

Although joint fluid is sent away for such studies as fungal and tuberculosis cultures, sugar concentration, and mucin clot testing, it is well to remember that probably the most immediately useful information is to be gleaned from the gross appearance of the fluid, a differential cell examination, Gram staining for bacteria, and inspection for urate and calcium pyrophosphate crystals. *These tests should be performed at once and by the operator himself.*

Synovial Biopsy

The Parker-Pearson synovial biopsy needle (Figure 3.12) is a superior instrument to the older, bulky Polley-Bickel trephine. It may be used in place of the standard 18-gauge aspirating needle after infiltration of the anesthetic agent. The 14-gauge outer sleeve, with stylet in place, is introduced into the joint in the usual manner, the stylet removed, and aspiration performed to confirm the position and to obtain a fluid specimen. With very few exceptions, the knee joint has been the site selected for biopsy.

The notched inner sleeve is now secured to the syringe and inserted into the outer cannula until it protrudes as illustrated in Figure 3.12. Suction is now applied again, both

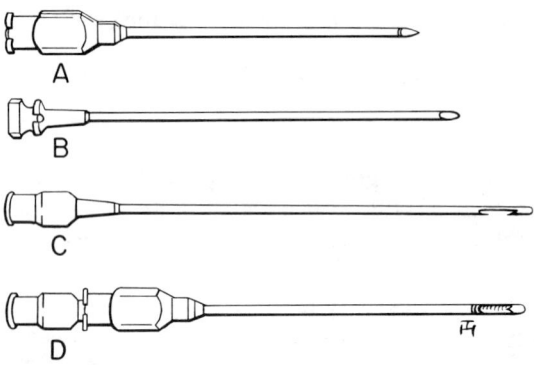

Figure 3.12.
Parker-Pearson synovial biopsy needle. (**A**) Outer sleeve. (**B**) Stylet. (**C**) Biopsy snare. (**D**) Biopsy snare in place in outer sleeve.

needles are slightly withdrawn, and after aspiration of a few milliliters of fluid, the redundant synovium will be sucked into the notch to plug it and prevent further return of fluid. *Suction is maintained on the syringe,* the inner sleeve is held motionless, and the outer cannula is advanced, with a slight twisting motion, for a distance of about 1 cm. This ensures that the specimen has been severed and held in the notch. The outer needle is left in place, and the inner one, with attached syringe, is removed. The amputated biopsy plug is teased from its notch with a needle onto filter paper, stretched (usually 2 to 5 mm length specimens are obtained), and fixed in 10% formalin. The entire process may be repeated frequently if necessary.

After the procedure is completed, the knee is wrapped with an elastic bandage after application of a dry dressing, and the patient is asked to remain at rest for 1 hour.

4.

BIOPSY TECHNIQUES

4.1. BONE MARROW ASPIRATION AND BIOPSY

Diagnostic bone marrow aspiration is performed commonly in two areas: the sternum, and both the anterior and posterior iliac crests. Sternal marrow is usually histologically superior, and should be aspirated first, with certain specific exceptions. The delicacy of the sternal architecture in infants, and the understandable terror engendered by a sternal aspiration in children, make the iliac crests, vertebral spines, or occasionally the tibia the preferred locations in the young. Fear of penetration through the sternum has led some authorities to recommend the iliac crests in cases of advanced osteoporosis or bleeding disorders. In fact, this complication is more often the result of carelessness than of pathologically soft bone. Sternal marrow aspirations should be supervised initially by experienced personnel. It should also be remembered that compression over the sternal puncture site will yield more effective local hemostasis than will compression over the deeper iliac crests. Hemophilia is generally accepted as a contraindication to either aspiration or biopsy of bone marrow.

Posterior superior iliac spine marrow biopsies are indicated in cases of granulomatous marrow infiltration, myelofibrosis, aplastic anemia, and malignant invasion, i.e., in those diseases in which marrow aspiration is likely to be inadequate, or has already proved so, or when cytoarchitecture is mandatory to establish the diagnosis.

MATERIAL

A sterilized marrow kit containing 16-gauge Rosenthal (Figure 4.1A) or Osgood needles, with obturators, in both the 1-inch and 2-inch lengths, 2 sterile towels, 25-gauge and 22-gauge needles, two 20-ml and three 5-ml syringes, 20 clean coverslips, 10 clean microscope slides, watch glass, ampules of local anesthetic, no. 11 scalpel blade and handle. Floor supplies: sterile gloves, antiseptic-soaked sponges, a specimen bottle with 10 percent formalin for clotted blood aspirates, and sterile culture tubes.

Comment. Also illustrated (Figure 4.1B) is a marrow aspiration needle with the Franseen point, Biers hub, and Luer-Lok obturator. The Luer-Lok makes it unnecessary to hold the obturator in place by pushing against it with the thumb during introduction through the skin—a common cause of overpenetration. The Westerman-Jensen needle for iliac spine biopsies (Figure 4.2) is in essence a modification of the basic Vim-Silverman needle, and is handled in precisely the same manner (see Section 4.2 for Vim-Silverman biopsy technique).

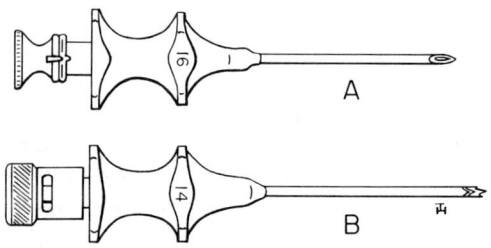

Figure 4.1.

Marrow aspiration needles. (**A**) Rosenthal needle and obturator. (**B**) Franseen point (serrated) needle. Luer-Lok obturator does not require thumb pressure to maintain its position during penetration of the skin and subcutaneous tissue.

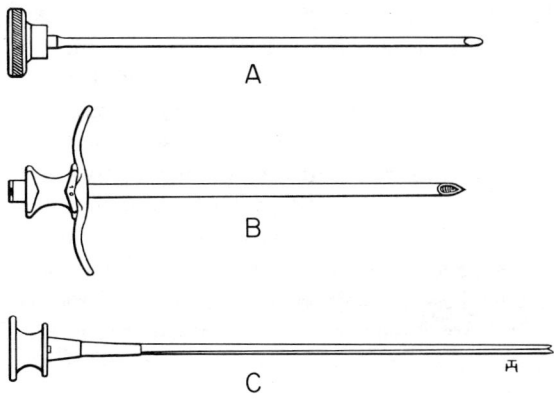

Figure 4.2.

Westerman-Jensen biopsy needle. (**A**) Obturator. (**B**) Outer sleeve. (**C**) Split inner sleeve.

TECHNIQUE

Both sternal and iliac crest aspirates are worthless if the smears and touch preparations are not properly handled. Should the physician doing the aspiration lack expertise in the preparation of marrow specimens, an experienced technician from either the pathology laboratory or the hematology laboratory should be present.

Sternal Marrow Aspiration

The patient is supine. This procedure may appear alarming to even the most nonchalant, and the steps should be explained in detail before beginning. An injection of 50 to 75 mg of Demerol prior to aspiration is an effective analgesic and sedative for the apprehensive patient. Also forewarn him that he will feel a sharp but brief pain during actual aspiration.

Select a midline spot at the level of the second interspace. Remember that the sternum is thinner, and thus the marrow more plentiful, between the interspaces than between the sternocostal junctions. If the index finger of the free hand is placed in the suprasternal notch, and the thumb and third finger in the second intercostal spaces, the center of the base of the triangle thus formed will mark the proper site for puncture. Wear gloves, prepare a wide area over the sternum, and drape with the towels. Infiltrate anesthesia along a tract that will allow the marrow needle to pass through the skin at a 45-degree angle and in a cephalad direction. Anesthetize the sensitive periosteum widely about the proposed site of puncture. Often this infiltrating needle will yield valuable information about the texture of the bone itself (soft and cheesy in myeloma, rock-hard in myelosclerosis). Pass the marrow needle with obturator in place along this tract, nicking the skin first with the scalpel blade if necessary. Use a firm, boring motion to advance only when the resistance of the bone is first encountered, then stop when a "give" is felt, indicating penetration of the marrow cavity.

This "give" may not be felt in a pathologic sternum, and is frequently not felt in iliac crest aspirations. In such cases, aspiration should be first attempted as soon as the needle is deep enough into cortex to be fixed in place. Remove the obturator and attach a 5-ml syringe to the hub of the needle. While this size is generally adequate, the 20-ml syringe may be required for additional suction, should the marrow prove hypercellular and thick. Apply firm, steady suction (warn the patient again that he will experience pain), until a few drops are aspirated, *but no more.* Remove the syringe and express the marrow, which will appear as whitish, granular particles, onto a slide or into the watch glass. Smears are made at once. Excessive initial suction will result only in dilution of the marrow by blood, but after the marrow is obtained, such diluted samples may be used for cultures, and clotted specimens fixed in Zenker's acetic acid solution or 10% formalin are useful for tumor cytology. Remove the needle and apply pressure over the puncture site for 5 minutes.

Should no marrow be aspirated on the first attempt, the obturator may be replaced and the needle advanced for a few millimeters for a second try. Repeatedly negative results, however, usually indicate that the sternal marrow is not suitable for aspiration. If only blood is obtained, a buffy coat preparation from it may be examined for abnormal cells.

Iliac Crest Aspiration and Biopsy

The patient will experience the same discomfort during suction that is felt during sternal aspiration, and he should be so warned. This pain is an important clue that the needle is actually within the marrow cavity.

For anterior iliac crest aspiration, the patient should lie on his side or be supine; for posterior iliac crest aspiration or spine biopsy, the patient is prone or on his side.

A spot approximately 2 cm inferior and posterior to the superior spine of the anterior crest is selected (Figure 4.3A). Preparation, infiltration, and aspiration are performed by a technique identical with that used for the sternum except that the longer marrow needle is used, and it passes through the skin at a right angle.

The posterior approach is usually selected for a Westerman-Jensen marrow biopsy. This large needle, with obturator properly seated, is passed through a nick in the skin and along an anesthetized tract that runs from directly behind the prominence of the posterior superior iliac spine (Figure 4.3B), and is at a right angle with the anterior abdominal wall. The physician will most comfortably be located behind the patient. The attached grip on the sleeve facilitates boring the needle into the spine until resistance abruptly yields, or until the needle is well embedded in the bone. The obturator is then removed, a few drops aspirated and made into smears, and the split inner cannula is introduced in a manner identical to that used with the Vim-Silverman needle. It is thrust straight into the marrow cavity, *without twisting.* This procedure is often quite painful. The outer sleeve is next advanced over the stationary cutting cannula, and both cannula and sleeve are twisted 180 degrees and removed as a unit. The specimen will be within the inner cannula. Imprints and proper fixation should be done immediately. The patient is instructed to lie on the side from

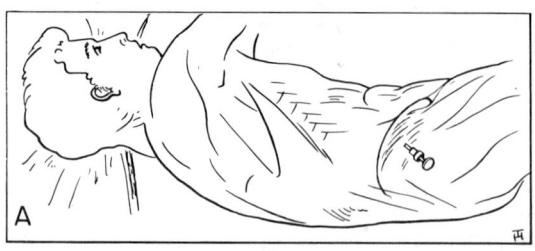

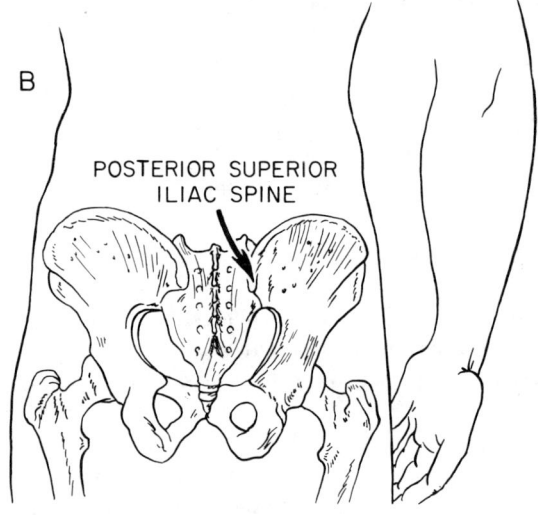

Figure 4.3.

(**A**) Needle position for anterior iliac crest aspiration. (**B**) Needle position for posterior superior iliac crest biopsy.

which the biopsy was taken, to effect hemostasis, and an order may be left for a mild analgesic.

Except for the extremely rare difficulty associated with inadvertent total penetration of the sternum, osteomyelitis is the single major complication following marrow biopsies, and is itself quite unusual. Careful aseptic technique should make it even more unusual. If both aspiration and needle biopsy are inadequate, the patient should be considered for an open sternal trephine biopsy.

4.2. VIM-SILVERMAN NEEDLE BIOPSY

At the bedside, the Vim-Silverman needle may be used to obtain biopsies of subcutaneous lymph nodes, breast masses, and deeper specimens from the liver. Since the use of this instrument in the former instance usually precedes surgical excision, placement of the puncture site should be such that both it and the penetration tract will be easily removed en bloc with the mass.

MATERIAL

A sterilized biopsy kit: 14-gauge Vim-Silverman needle, ampules of local anesthetic, 25-gauge and 22-gauge needles, 5-ml syringe, no. 11 scalpel blade and handle, skin stitches, forceps, towels. Floor supplies: sterile gloves, antiseptic-soaked sponges, dry dressings, sterile saline solution, filter paper, 10% formalin in biopsy jars.

Comment. The needle is in three parts (Figure 4.4): outer sleeve, stylet, and split inner, or cutting, sleeve. Before using the needle, test all three components for proper fit.

TECHNIQUE

Wearing gloves, prepare the skin widely over the mass and drape off the area. Infiltrate the proposed puncture site with anesthetic, but avoid actual penetration of the lesion with the needle, depositing the solution above, around, and if feasible, beneath it. Nick the skin to allow free passage of the biopsy needle, then advance the outer sleeve, with the stylet in place, until the point has penetrated the mass. Mobile lesions must actually be impaled before using the split inner sleeve, or they will be simply pushed away and no specimen obtained. Remove the stylet and place it next to the inner cannula to judge the point on the latter where it will begin to protrude beyond the end of the outer sleeve. The cannula may be grasped with the forceps at this spot.

Pass this cutting sleeve through the outer sleeve until this point is reached or resistance is felt. Hold the outer sleeve stable while the split cannula is next thrust into the lesion, to its full length if possible. *Do not twist the inner cannula as it is advanced.* Now grasp the inner cannula so that it

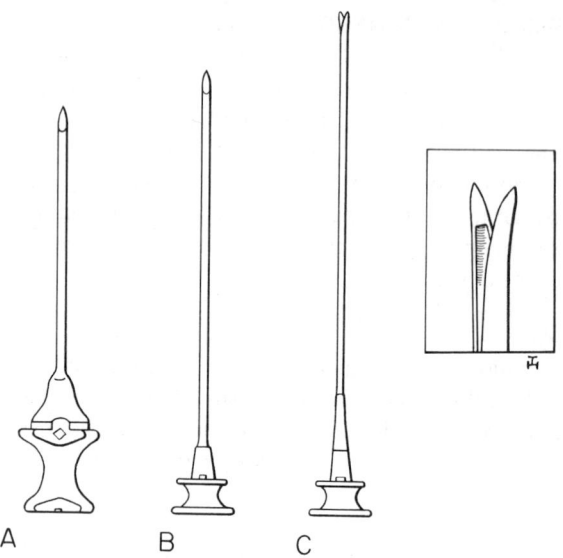

Figure 4.4.

Vim-Silverman biopsy needle. (**A**) Outer sleeve. (**B**) Stylet. (**C**) Split inner cutting cannula. Inset: Franklin modification with solid tabs to pinch off biopsy specimen.

remains stationary, and push the outer sleeve down over it until the tips of the two sleeves are again approximated. It is the shearing action of the passage of this outer sleeve that separates the biopsy. If the inner cannula has the Franklin modification (inset, Figure 4.4), the flattened tabs at the tip will cut off the core of tissue; if not, twist both inner and outer sleeves, as a single unit, 180 degrees before withdrawing. During the penetration passage of the inner cannula and also the second advancement of the outer cannula, it may be necessary to stabilize the lesion with the free hand, particularly if the lesion has a fibrous feel and is mobile. As the needle is withdrawn, be careful to maintain the relative positions of the two sleeves.

Apply 5 minutes of pressure over the puncture site. Free the biopsy core from the inner cannula with a needle onto a moistened piece of filter paper and examine it for adequacy.

Fix at once in formalin. A stitch may be used to close the incision, and a dry dressing applied.

4.3. NEEDLE BIOPSY OF THE LIVER

Although not totally obviating the need for occasional open liver biopsies, the success of the percutaneous needle biopsy in properly selected patients should make this the first technique considered when the differential diagnosis of liver disease requires tissue histology. The following criteria will help to increase the percentage of successful biopsies and reduce the incidence of complications.

1. When the intercostal route is chosen, the patient must be able to hold his breath to prevent a possible tear in the hepatic capsule. Unconscious or confused patients are, therefore, not ideal candidates for this approach. In infants (and to a less successful degree in adults), the chest may be stabilized by external compression after expiration.

2. Because the major complication following needle biopsy is hemorrhage, bleeding parameters must be checked and improved if necessary. AquaMEPHYTON (Vitamin K_1) may be used to improve the Quick prothrombin time; if the patient is severely jaundiced, 10 mg should be given 48 hours prior to biopsy even when the prothrombin time is normal. Inability to raise the prothrombin percentage above 50 is a contraindication to needle biopsy. Many patients, moreover, have associated conditions, such as uremia, that can lead to first-stage clotting defects not detected by the Quick prothrombin time; the screening usefulness of the standard bleeding and clotting times, though crude, can often lead to the diagnosis and treatment of unsuspected deficiencies. The platelet count should be over 75,000.

3. The presence of ascites, while not an absolute contraindication for biopsy, does make the procurement of an adequate sample difficult by allowing the surface of the liver to float away from the tip of the advancing needle. The fluid should, therefore, first be tapped or decreased with

diuretics, and if some persists, the patient should be biopsied in a semisitting position. When the intercostal route is employed, pleural fluid also should first be removed. Infection in the pleural cavity rules out this approach.

4. Small livers can be missed entirely by the needle. The use of a plain film of the abdomen and chest prior to biopsy (for fluid and the position of the right hemidiaphragm) should be standard. A liver scan will yield a more accurate representation of organ size, and may also demonstrate unsuspected lesions that will alter the biopsy approach.

5. The patient should have nothing but liquids for 12 hours prior to biopsy, and a mild sedative, such as 150 mg of Nembutal, may be given 30 minutes before the procedure if he is restless. Two units of blood should be cross-matched and available.

MATERIAL

A sterilized liver biopsy kit: Menghini needle in the standard 1.6-mm diameter, skin-piercing stylet or no. 11 scalpel blade, two 5-ml syringes, ampules of local anesthetic, 25-gauge and 20-gauge needles, 22-gauge spinal needle, gauze sponges. Floor supplies: sterile saline solution, antiseptic-soaked sponges, sterile gloves, filter paper, and 10% formalin in biopsy jars.

Comment. The Menghini needle (Figure 4.5) has a slightly oblique tip and an edge that is beveled on the outside, allowing a good biopsy cut without rotation. It will not pierce skin and tough fibrous tissue and it should not be used to do so; it should be sharpened after each biopsy. In addition, it is fitted with a nail or angulated stopping plug that allows fluid to pass back and forth around it, and that transmits suction from the syringe to the needle tip, but that will not enter the syringe on suction because of the head or the bend, and thus will not allow the biopsy specimen to be inadvertently aspirated through the needle into the barrel of the syringe. As shown in the illustration, the needle may also be fitted with a device to limit its depth of penetration.

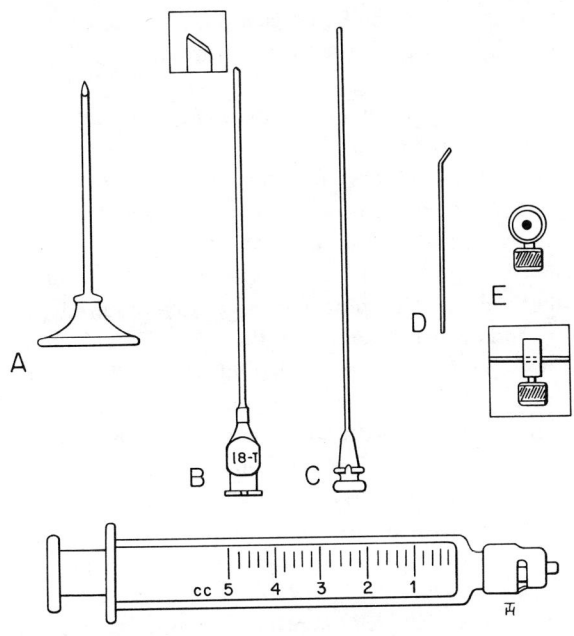

Figure 4.5.

Menghini needle. (**A**) Skin-piercing stylet. (**B**) Biopsy needle. (**C**) Obturator. (**D**) Stopping plug. (**E**) Depth-limiting attachment.

TECHNIQUE

The first biopsy should be attempted with the help of an experienced physician.

Intercostal Approach

This is generally the most satisfactory route, for it presents the full depth of the right lobe of the liver for penetration and avoids abdominal viscera. The pleural space, however, is transversed.

The patient lies supine in bed, close to its right edge, with his trunk tilted slightly to the right by a pillow beneath his left side. His right arm rests behind his head, and the face is turned to the left. The site chosen is usually the ninth or tenth intercostal space in the midaxillary line, but the precise location is determined by percussion, and is one interspace below the point of maximum dullness during expiration.

Gloves are worn. The lateral thorax is widely cleansed and draped. Anesthetic is infiltrated along the proposed biopsy tract, which will pass immediately above the rib forming the lower border of the selected interspace, and which will penetrate the pleura, diaphragm, peritoneum, and finally the liver capsule. Each of these structures should be anesthetized, and the spinal needle may be required for the pleura and deeper structures in the obese. To prevent rents in the liver capsule during deep infiltration, have the patient hold his breath in expiration until the needle is withdrawn. The biopsy path will be such as to pass at right angles through the diaphragm, and thus will be slightly inferiorly and anteriorly directed, roughly along an imaginary line from the site of the skin puncture through the umbilicus. A nick is made in the skin with the piercing stylet or scalpel blade.

The 5-ml syringe will give the proper degree of suction. Fill it with 3 ml of sterile saline solution, connect it with the Menghini needle after the bent stopping plug is inserted, and advance the needle along the tract to, but not through, the intercostal space (Figure 4.6). Inject 2 ml of fluid to clear the needle and then ask the patient to hold his breath in expiration. Apply suction to the syringe and maintain it; then, in a single motion, rapidly transverse the pleura and penetrate the diaphragm and liver. There will be a palpable "give" as the diaphragm is punctured, and the needle guard may be preset to prevent overly deep penetration in thin individuals. No rotation is required, and the needle is immediately extracted while still under aspiration. The tip is placed in the formalin solution, suction is released for the first time, and a small amount of saline solution is expelled to free the biopsy, if necessary. The trocar may also be used to push out the core of tissue.

Cirrhotic, fibrotic biopsies are likely to fragment in the formalin jars, and if cirrhosis is suspected, the tissue cylinder should be gently expelled onto moistened filter paper or

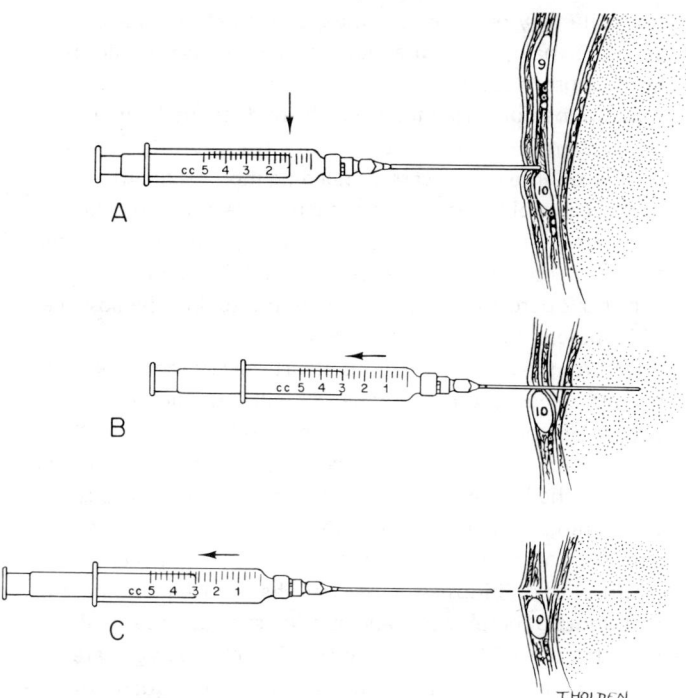

Figure 4.6.

Technique of Menghini needle biopsy of the liver. (**A**) Needle advanced to intercostal space. (**B**) Needle plunged into liver parenchyma while suction is applied to the syringe, and the patient holds his breath in expiration. (**C**) Immediate removal of needle while suction is maintained.

lens paper, then placed directly into the perforated plastic "boats" used for fixation by the pathology department.

Should no satisfactory specimen be obtained, a new tract may be anesthetized, using the same skin perforation. Only a single repeat effort is recommended by most authorities.

Postbiopsy, the patient lies on his right side for two hours, and is placed on bed-rest and a 2-hour chart for the next 24-hour period. This is an important precaution inasmuch as many of the cases of hemorrhage do not occur or manifest themselves until 12 or more hours have passed. The patient normally may be expected to experience some local or epigastric pain, often of a pleuritic nature, and should be given appropriate analgesia.

Severe hemorrhage may occur from distended hepatic veins, aberrant arteries, a tear in the liver capsule, or, rarely, an injured intercostal vessel. Bleeding most frequently complicates biopsies in patients with severe hepatocellular disease rather than obstructive disease, and usually responds to transfusion and thoracentesis. Overall incidence is low, about 0.2 percent, and is extremely unusual in the absence of jaundice.

Despite the most meticulous efforts, every individual who performs these biopsies frequently will cause an occasional case of bile peritonitis. This may be produced by puncture of the gallbladder or by penetration of a distended bile duct beneath the liver capsule. Although the intercostal route will diminish the incidence of the former, bile lakes are almost impossible to avoid and have led, in some centers, to a refusal to do biopsies in cases of obstructive jaundice. In fact, most punctures seal and subside spontaneously, although a few will require drainage. The clinical signs are those of chemical peritonitis, with right upper quadrant pain, tenderness, and rigor. Chills and fever may also be encountered, particularly if there is bacterial growth in the bile.

Right shoulder pain rather commonly follows this technique, and is secondary either to the diaphragmatic irritation caused by a small amount of hepatic bleeding, or to a small pneumothorax. A significant air leak is rare with the Menghini needle biopsy, but it does occasionally occur when the Vim-Silverman needle is used. The technique for liver biopsy with this instrument is precisely the same as that described in Section 4.2, Vim-Silverman Needle Biopsy, using the intercostal route outlined here. The core obtained is larger and is, therefore, less likely to fall apart when the biopsy is cirrhotic; however, the technique is slower and more cumbersome, and the incidence of complications is increased.

Inadvertent biopsies of the colon and kidney have been reported, but they are rarely dangerous.

Subcostal Approach

This route may be chosen only when the liver is grossly enlarged three fingerbreadths below the costal margin and is easily palpable. Its main advantage lies in the ability to biopsy individual lesions. For a nonspecific puncture of the right hepatic lobe, the skin is pierced to the right of the xyphoid process in the midclavicular line, and the needle is directed toward the tip of the right shoulder into the bulk of the lobe and away from the hilar structures.

4.4. PLEURAL BIOPSY

The primary indication for pleural biopsy is recurrent, unexplained pleural effusion; its greatest usefulness is in the diagnosis of tuberculosis. A malignant effusion whose etiology has remained obscure after standard pleural fluid examinations may also yield to this technique, but the patchy nature of most pleural metastases makes this the exception rather than the rule. Collagen diseases involving the pleura may also occasionally be identified by biopsy. Preparation and contraindications are the same as for thoracentesis, and the section on this subject should be reviewed before beginning. To avoid a visceral pleural or pulmonary biopsy, this procedure should not be attempted in the absence of demonstrable fluid by x-ray.

MATERIAL

All the material required for a thoracentesis (see Section 3.1) should be available, plus biopsy jars filled with 10% formalin. The Cope pleural biopsy needle (Figure 4.7) should be checked for proper fit of all components before beginning this procedure. An assistant is required, and the first biopsy should be performed under experienced guidance.

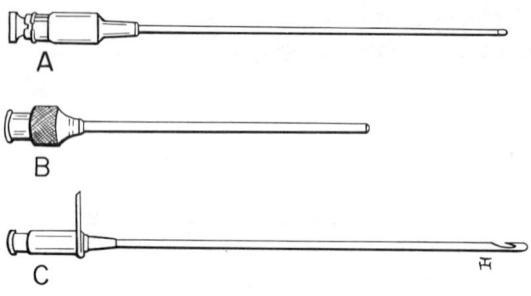

Figure 4.7.

Cope biopsy needle. (**A**) Inner needle with stylet. (**B**) Outer sleeve. (**C**) Biopsy snare.

TECHNIQUE

The patient is positioned and prepared for a lateral thoracentesis (see Figure 3.1). Because his cooperation in breathing is required to avoid a possible pneumothorax, he should be reasonably alert and able to take deep, slow breaths. Gloves are worn. An anesthetic wheal is raised in the mid- or posterior axillary line, over the interspace appropriate for the fluid level. The pleura should be widely anesthetized. The outer sleeve of the Cope needle is 11 gauge, and a nick in the skin will be necessary to allow its passage. Pass the 13-gauge inner puncture needle with its fitted stylet through this outer sleeve; it should fit snugly and protrude slightly. The pleura is now entered as for a standard thoracentesis, care being taken to pass immediately above the selected rib.

When it is estimated that the pleural cavity has been entered, the patient is asked to take a deep breath and then exhale slowly through pursed lips, so that he may be heard by the operator. While he is doing this, the stylet is removed; if the pleural space has been entered, a free flow of fluid will be seen. This maneuver must be accomplished before the patient inhales to avoid a pneumothorax. The stylet is then reinserted. The patient is again asked to exhale slowly, the inner needle and stylet are removed, and a thumb is placed over the opening of the outer sleeve. The hook-tipped curette, with the stylet inserted in it by the assistant, is slid into the outer sleeve, the patient again exhaling slowly until the needle is in position.

The pleura may be biopsied anywhere *along a downward-directed arc of 180 degrees.* Biopsies taken upward are contraindicated because of potential injury to the neurovascular bundle beneath the superior adjacent rib. An indicator on the handle of the curette points in the same direction as the hook, to allow biopsy in a specific position. After full insertion, the curette is slowly withdrawn until the pleura is snared, and resistance is felt. The outer sleeve is steadied with the free hand, and then pushed forward, while traction is exerted on the biopsy snare. The beveled edge of the outer sleeve transects the specimen. As the biopsy is withdrawn, the outer sleeve remains in place, and the patient is again asked to exhale slowly. A finger is placed over the open end of the outer sleeve, while the biopsy snare is passed to the assistant, who frees the tissue plug and fixes it at once in formalin. The stylet is now removed from the biopsy snare needle, and the latter is fitted to a three-way stopcock and 50-cc syringe combination for a standard thoracentesis. To avoid excessive fluid leakage through the rent in the parietal pleura, the patient should be "tapped dry," if feasible, or up to an arbitrary limit of 1200–1500 cc.

Prior to removal of the needle, a second biopsy may be taken from a different quadrant. After the specimen has been transected, curette, syringe, and outer sleeve are withdrawn as a single unit. The patient is requested to lie for two hours on the side opposite that biopsied, to further minimize fluid leakage. A chest film is obtained following each biopsy to ascertain the presence or absence of a pneumothorax.

Note. When sending pleural biopsy specimens to the pathology laboratory, be certain that their origin is clearly indicated, as well as the suspected diagnosis.

4.5. COLLECTION OF CYTOLOGY SPECIMENS

Properly obtained, properly prepared, and properly studied cytologic specimens have proved a valuable adjunct in the early diagnosis of malignancy in selected organs. A good yield of information depends, however, not only on the physician's ability to present the pathologist with suitable specimens, but also on the latter's experience and ability to interpret them. The following instructions will keep the physician's role in this cooperative effort functioning properly; however, it is wise first to sound out the pathology department, particularly on the more specialized exfoliative techniques, to ascertain their interest and proficiency in reading the specimens.

Barr Sex Chromatin Mass

Determination of sex chromatin mass can be made by a study of cells from either the buccal or the vaginal mucosa.

Buccal mucosa
The mucosa from the inside of the cheek should be scraped firmly but not deeply with a tongue blade. The material is spread onto a clean glass slide and immersed at once in Papanicolaou fixative.

Vaginal Mucosa
The lateral wall of the vagina is scraped firmly with a tongue blade. The material is spread onto a clean glass slide and placed at once in Papanicolaou fixative.

Cerebrospinal Fluid

After the fluid is collected, 2 to 5 ml or more should be brought to the cytology laboratory as soon as possible. If any delay occurs, the fluid should be refrigerated without addition of any preservative.

Oral Mucosa

Scrape the lesion vigorously with a tongue blade. If the surface is dry, apply saline solution before scraping. Smear material from the tongue blade over two-thirds of the slide, and place it immediately in Papanicolaou fixative.

Breast Secretions

Every breast disorder associated with an areolar discharge should have cytologic studies of the fluid. A clean slide should be placed in contact with the nipple and the material collected on it.

The slide should *never* be air-dried; a second slide should be placed over the first and then pulled apart. The slides are then separated with a paper clip and immersed in Papanicolaou fixative. If fluid is aspirated from a breast cyst, it should be brought in the fresh state at once to the cytology laboratory for processing.

Respiratory Tract

Early morning deep cough specimens are best for examination, and three to five separate collections should be sent. The sputum should be sent to the cytology laboratory while very fresh, or fixed on slides as follows:

1. Samples should be selected from the specimen with a tongue blade, and should include yellow or white flecks, or areas with blood.

2. Two-thirds of a slide with a paper clip on one end is gently smeared and fixed in Papanicolaou solution immediately.

The use of a paper clip prevents two slides in the same bottle from becoming adherent to each other, and such a clip should be used whenever more than one slide is sent.

If the patient is unable to produce adequate amounts of sputum, the use of a water aerosol, delivered by a positive pressure respirator or ultrasonic nebulizer, may assist in bringing up useful samples. This must be done immediately prior to collection and directed by those experienced with the apparatus.

During prebronchoscopic anesthesia and the examination itself, all secretions coughed up or aspirated should be spread at once by the method above. In addition, the yield will be increased by submitting *fresh* all secretions expectorated in the first 24 hours following bronchoscopy.

Pleural, Peritoneal, and Pericardial Fluids

Optimum results will be achieved through a double examination: Papanicolaou smears and cell block examination. A single specimen of 100 to 200 ml will suffice for both tests, although smaller amounts should also be submitted. No preservatives should be added to the specimen, although it may be refrigerated overnight if necessary. Oxalate is used to counteract any tendency of the fluid to clot.

Esophageal Washings

Obtain the samples after an 8-hour period of fasting to prevent regurgitation of food. As outlined in Chapter 8, Nasogastric Intubation, pass a Levin tube (preferably plastic) in the usual manner, but stop the tube in the esophagus, usually a distance of between 35 and 40 cm. Have the patient swallow normal saline solution while simultaneously aspirating the tube gently, and save this fluid in a container placed in an iced bath. Lavage the esophagus with 40 ml of saline solution, withdraw, and repeat until about 100 ml of wash has been placed in a second container in the iced bath. Advance the tube into the stomach, aspirate the additional fluid but label it separately, and send all collections at once to the cytology laboratory.

Gastric Washings

Specimens for cytologic examination should be obtained before, or at least 24 hours after, any barium study by mouth. Food and fluids except water should be withheld for 12 hours prior to the collection.

A Levin tube (preferably plastic) is passed into the stomach by the method described in Chapter 8. Any material in the stomach is aspirated and either discarded or labeled separately. Three hundred ml of saline wash are instilled into the stomach and forcefully barbotaged back and forth. This fluid is aspirated completely and placed into a bottle labeled "1" in an iced bath. Four hundred ml of saline solution are again instilled into the stomach, and the patient is turned onto his right side, back, and left side for two minutes each while the fluid is continuously barbotaged. All this is again aspirated and placed into a second bottle marked "2," and both containers are sent *at once* to the cytology laboratory.

Colonic Washings

Success in this technique requires thorough cleansing of the colon prior to the examination. Two ounces of a sodium phosphate oral cathartic, or one-half can of X-Prep by mouth the evening prior to the day of the washing, has been generally satisfactory. On the morning of the procedure, elevate the foot of the bed on 12-inch blocks and administer saline-solution enemas with the patient on his left side. In this position, most individuals are able to retain from 2,500 to 3,500 ml of fluid per enema, and four or five enemas are sufficient to cleanse the colon. The patient turns on his back, then onto his right side before expelling the enema. The final return must contain no particulate matter and should be absolutely clear. An hour's wait following this final enema, before starting the cytology test, ensures a better cell collection.

Intubation
Introduce a proctoscope as far as possible, with the patient in the Sims position, and pass a no. 12 French red rubber catheter a few centimeters beyond the end of the proctoscope. Withdraw the proctoscope and instill 1,000 ml of

saline solution slowly through the catheter. Turn the patient supine and massage the abdomen vigorously, wait several minutes, and collect the irrigating solution.

The wash is collected in a 1,000-ml beaker that is immersed in ice water. From this beaker, the fluid is poured through a strainer into 50-ml centrifuge tubes, centrifuged for 2 minutes, and then processed. The same procedure is then repeated, using 800 ml of sodium acetate buffer (pH 5.5), instead of the saline solution.

Female Genital Tract

Douching or bathing even several hours before the smear is taken, or a preliminary manual examination with lubricant, will alter the true histology of the secretions, and these measures should be avoided.

A nonlubricated speculum (or one moistened by warm water) is inserted and the entire cervix is scraped with an Ayre spatula or longitudinally split tongue blade. These instruments are superior to cotton applicator sticks. The material is smeared at once on a slide and immersed in Papanicolaou fixative. An aspirator on a syringe is then introduced into the cervical canal, suction applied, and the material then ejected onto a slide, smeared evenly, and fixed in Papanicolaou solution.

Cell readings suspicious for either adenocarcinoma of the uterus or squamous cell carcinoma of the cervix should be followed up by endometrial biopsies in the first instance, and cervical punch biopsies or cone biopsy in the latter instance.

A vaginal smear for hormonal evaluation is obtained by scraping the lateral wall of the vagina with a tongue blade or spatula. The material is spread evenly over a slide and immersed at once in Papanicolaou fixative.

The first voided morning specimen is preferred for evaluation of ovarian steroid production. A fresh specimen may be sent to the laboratory within two hours, but if a longer delay is probable, the urine should be added to a bottle containing 30 ml of 70% alcohol.

Urine

In evaluation for malignant cells, a freshly voided specimen or one obtained by catheter should be brought promptly to the cytology laboratory for smear preparation. A concentrated first-morning specimen is optimum.

5.

ENDOSCOPY

5.1. INDIRECT LARYNGOSCOPY

Indirect laryngoscopy is an integral part of every physical examination of a patient with symptoms referable to the hypopharynx and larynx. It should also precede any elective bronchoscopy. A firm but sympathetic approach to the patient, and a careful explanation of the procedure prior to starting it, have been shown repeatedly to reduce the incidence of the gagging that can make this examination impossible.

MATERIAL
Head mirror, no. 5 laryngeal mirror (the standard size for adults), gooseneck lamp, alcohol lamp, gauze sponges. For topical anesthesia 4% Xylocaine or 1% Pontocaine may be used, but in general this is not necessary.
Comment. The head mirror should ride comfortably on the forehead, so that it does not slip during the examination, and it must come well down over the left eye, close enough to it to touch the skin or glasses. Close the right eye and focus the beam on the patient's face to a small brilliant spot. Remember that the fixed focal length of the mirror means that the only method of maintaining brightness

throughout the examination is for the operator to move his head back and forth appropriately.

TECHNIQUE

The position and comfort of both examiner and patient during this examination are important. The patient should sit erect with his chin forward, his feet on the floor, and his head free to move. The doctor must be comfortably seated, with his head approximately on the same level as that of the patient. A gooseneck lamp should be positioned behind the patient's right ear and at the level of his head.

The patient is asked to stick out his tongue, and then a gauze is placed over it and wrapped under it, to prevent wadding on the surface of the tongue from becoming a visual obstruction, and also to protect the undersurface of the tongue against the sharp lower incisor teeth. The tongue is grasped lightly between the left thumb and middle finger, and the index finger is braced against the patient's upper lip or upper teeth. If the patient does not pull back his tongue, the examiner will find it unnecessary to exert actual traction on it. The flame of the alcohol lamp is directed against the surface of the mirror to warm it and then the back side of the mirror is tested against the hand for warmth. An excellent alternative to this method is to dip the mirror in undiluted pHisoHex before beginning the examination and then wipe it dry. The mirror will remain completely free of fogging for the entire examination.

Hold the mirror midway along the shaft, like a pen, and not by the handle. The fingers are braced against the patient's cheek, and the mirror is inserted in the mouth so that the edge advances with the glass surface flush with the tongue. This means that it is not introduced in its greatest diameter. The back side of the mirror is then rested against the uvula, and it and the soft palate are swept upward and backward in a single gentle motion. Once contact with the uvula is made, the mirror is not shifted to any great extent, although slight movement may be necessary to visualize the full larynx. In general, gagging is not caused by contact with the uvula and soft palate, but rather by touching the posterior surface of the tongue or the posterior wall of the pharynx. Remember that anterior and posterior relations as seen by the mirror are reversed, whereas right and left remain the same.

The patient is asked to breathe quietly through the mouth, and should be told firmly that as long as he does so he will not gag. Patients who are "gaggers" are sometimes eased by being told to "pant through the mouth like a dog." After initial examination and during a period of quiet respirations, the patient is asked to sound a high-pitched "e-e-e-e-e," or better, "he-e-e-e-e." *The phonation must be high-pitched and prolonged.* It is best if the operator demonstrates the sound he wishes and actually accompanies the patient. Make sure the light remains in focus at all times.

The hypopharynx is examined first, including the circumvallate papillae, lingual tonsils, valecullae, and epiglottis. This final structure is drawn anteriorly when the patient phonates the high pitched "e-e-e-e-e," allowing visualization of the anterior portion of the vocal cords.

When examining the larynx (Figure 5.1), the operator should not fix his attention only on the true cords. He should also observe the false cords, the arytenoid cartilages, and the laryngeal ventricle (the space directly beneath the false cords, best seen by having the patient tilt his head sideways). The pyriform recesses lie posterior and lateral to the arytenoid cartilages, and they will dilate slightly if the patient says "a-a-a-a-a" in a low voice. Examine the larynx both in quiet respiration and during phonation. Adequate phonation usually reveals the anterior commissure of the true cords, the most difficult portion to visualize during indirect laryngoscopy.

5.2. BEDSIDE BRONCHOSCOPY

As an emergency procedure, bedside bronchoscopy is an invaluable therapeutic technique. It is clearly indicated in the urgent treatment of vomiting with aspiration, overwhelming pulmonary secretions associated with broncho-

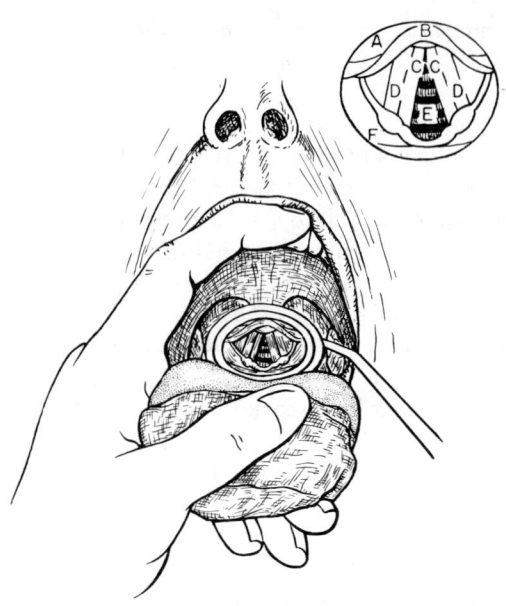

Figure 5.1.

Both patient and examiner should be comfortably seated for indirect laryngoscopy. The tongue is grasped with a gauze and held forward gently. The back of the mirror is rested against the uvula and soft palate. Care is taken not to touch the sensitive posterior wall of the pharynx or posterior surface of the tongue. Inset: Laryngeal structures as seen in the mirror: **A**, vallecula; **B**, epiglottis; **C**, true vocal cords; **D**, false vocal cords; **E**, trachea; **F**, arytenoid cartilage.

pneumonia, and massive postoperative atelectasis. In the management of such cases of respiratory distress, however, bronchoscopy should be thought of as a part of a graded therapeutic response, one that will include chest physical therapy and endotracheal suction at one end of the scale of severity, and emergency tracheostomy at the other. Bedside bronchoscopy is not meant to replace elective diagnostic examination, nor is it adequate for this task.

MATERIAL

Sterilized bronchoscopy kit: Jackson 8 mm × 40 cm bronchoscope with long-handled light carrier, suction tip, sponge forceps and biopsy forceps, 1 Luken's tube with stopper and rubber connector (Figure 5.2), 1 cross-action laryngeal

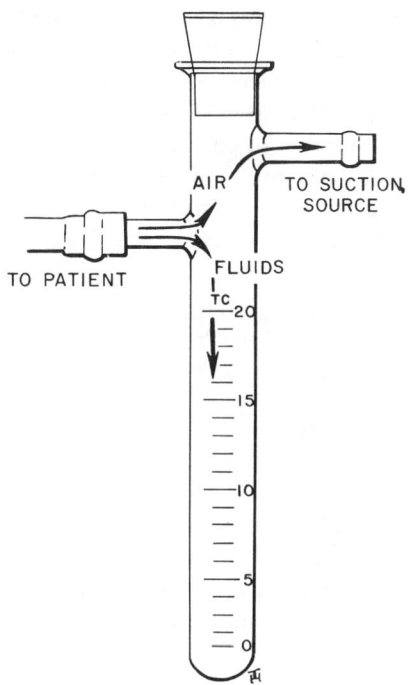

Figure 5.2.

Luken's tube. Fluid aspirated from the patient collects in the bottom of the tube and is easily removed for diagnostic studies.

forceps, 4 towel clips, 2 Luer-Lok 10-ml syringes, 2 catheter adapter tips, 1 small solution basin, suction tubing, light cord, 4 towels, and gauze sponges. Floor supplies: cotton pledgets, culture tubes, oxygen tubing, laryngoscope, topical anesthetic in an atomizer, sterile saline solution for irrigation, sterile gloves, masks, and gowns.

Note. A battery box should accompany the bronchoscopy kit, and the bronchoscope light should be tested before beginning. An Ambu bag with face mask and oral airway should be available.

TECHNIQUE

The patient, who will usually be in respiratory distress, should be lying supine along the edge of the bed with the mattress elevated 45 degrees to ease his breathing. His head should also be at the top edge of the mattress, with a folded blanket or pillow beneath his shoulders to allow slight extension of the neck (Figure 5.3). The operator stands either at the corner of the mattress or on a stool behind the headboard. It may prove more comfortable to sit on the headboard. A nurse or assistant must be in attendance. Supplemental oxygen should be continued until immediately prior to passage of the bronchoscope. Briefly explain the nature of the procedure and its rationale.

Wear gloves and mask. Protect the patient's eyes with a towel, and if he wears dentures, remove them. Topical anesthesia of the entire oropharynx is accomplished via a thorough spraying with 3 to 4 ml of 0.5% Pontocaine, or 4% Xylocaine. Although Xylocaine is less likely to cause the idiosyncratic reaction seen occasionally with Pontocaine, it is slightly less effective as a topical anesthetic agent. Adherence to the volumes suggested should avoid trouble, but the operator must be prepared to handle an untoward reaction such as a convulsion; this frequently requires endo-

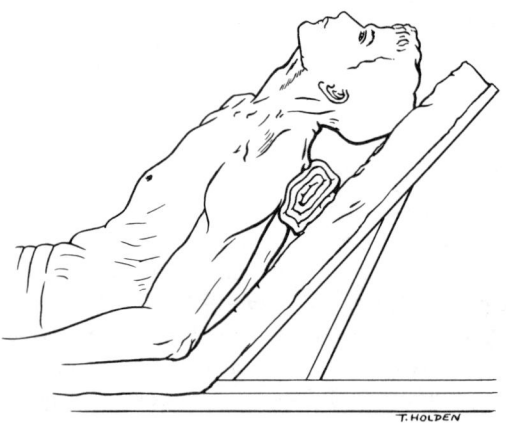

Figure 5.3.

Patient position for bedside bronchoscopy. If the towel does not allow for sufficient extension of the neck, the head may be held by an assistant over the end of the mattress.

tracheal intubation and intravenous barbiturate sedation. A small cotton pledget, dipped into the anesthetic solution and held by the cross-action laryngeal forceps, may be guided into each vallecula for additional anesthesia. Finally, the vocal cords may be visualized with the laryngoscope and briefly sprayed. Inasmuch as an intact cough reflex is important, deeper anesthesia is not indicated.

A gauze sponge is fitted over the upper lip to protect it. Rest the left hand on this sponge, with the bronchoscope lying across the thumb, and the middle finger retracting the upper lip from the teeth; the thumb will act as a fulcrum for the bronchoscope (Figure 5.4). Holding the bronchoscope handle upward (lip anterior), between the thumb and index finger of the right hand, enter the right side of the mouth and pass the bronchoscope over the tongue until the

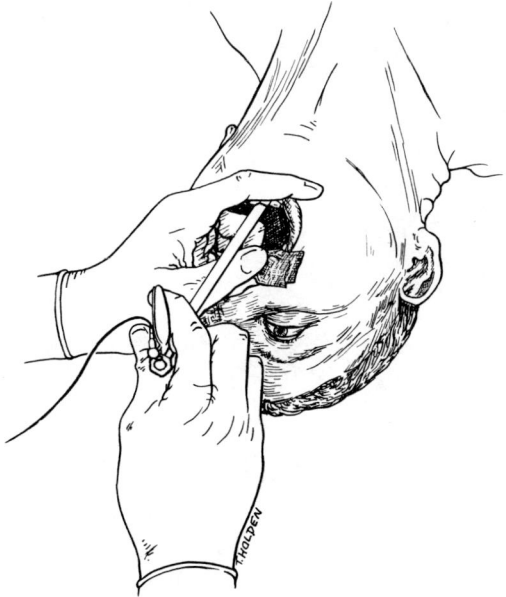

Figure 5.4.

Introduction of the bronchoscope. Note that the instrument rests on the left thumb, and that this digit serves as the fulcrum, also protecting the patient's upper teeth. The left middle finger retracts the upper lip from the teeth.

epiglottis comes into view. The larynx and vocal cords will be seen when the epiglottis is lifted anteriorly with the tip of the bronchoscope. Do this by depressing the proximal end held by the right hand, using the left thumb both as a fulcrum and as protection for the front teeth (Figure 5.5). With the handle to the right direct the aperture of the bronchoscope at the left vocal cord, thus bringing the lip of the instrument through the center of the gap between the two cords. Once through, turn the handle upward. Difficulty passing the larynx may often be relieved by flexing the patient's neck, thus bringing the axis of the larynx into a line with that of the oral cavity. An assistant may also push the larynx into view by pressing inward on the neck over it.

After a brief inspection of the vocal cords, the bronchoscope is passed into the trachea. The neck may be extended over the edge of the bed if necessary, with the head held by an assistant, to avoid the obstruction of prominent upper teeth. Turning the head to either the left or right will help to direct the instrument into the opposite mainstem bron-

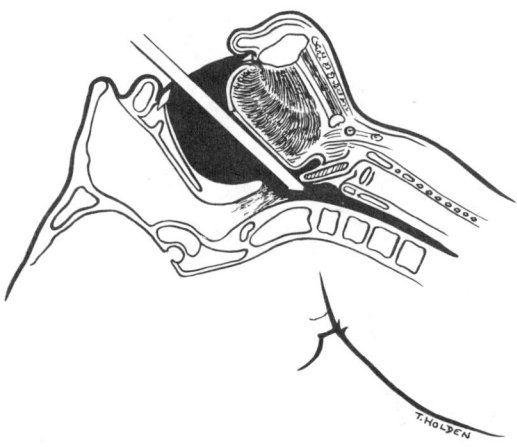

Figure 5.5.

Passage of the bronchoscope. The tip of the instrument is levered upward at this point by depressing the proximal end and rocking it on the left thumb as a fulcrum. This elevates the epiglottis and allows visualization of the vocal cords.

chus. Guide the tube with the left hand. Vigorous coughing and gagging during this period may further decrease the patient's oxygenation. The use of supplemental oxygen via the side arm of the bronchoscope, both during intubation and between periods of suctioning, can avoid potential disaster.

The operator must also be ready to deal with laryngospasm occurring during his attempts at intubation. The bronchoscope should be removed, and respiration should be assisted if necessary with an oral airway and an Ambu bag. Inspiratory pressure should be so delivered as to coincide with the patient's own respiratory efforts. Bronchospasm will usually respond to bronchodilators and, if not contraindicated, increased sedation.

Secretions blocking the trachea are aspirated first, using the Luken's tube (see Figure 5.2), to facilitate sputum collection for culture or cytology. Each mainstem bronchus is next suctioned clear until secondary orifices are visualized (Figure 5.6). Repeated irrigations of 5 to 10 ml of sterile saline solution or dilute Mucomyst solution (acetylcysteine) are used to lavage the tracheobronchial tree after aspiration of vomitus or to clear inspissated secretions.

When removing a foreign body with the biopsy forceps, the thumb and ring finger are passed through the handle rings, the middle finger is wrapped around the handle shaft, and the index finger is laid perpendicular along the handle shaft. This manner enables the operator to determine with the index finger the position of the forceps blades and to exert traction *with this finger alone, along a direct line with the bronchial lumen,* when the object is removed. After grasping the foreign body, the forceps is withdrawn to the tip of the bronchoscope, and then both are removed as a single unit.

The patient is not allowed oral intake until the topical anesthesia has dissipated, usually 2 to 3 hours. Chest physical therapy combined with inhalation therapy can greatly enhance the effectiveness of bronchoscopy, if performed vigorously during the first 12 hours after intubation. X-rays are important aids in determining the results of therapy.

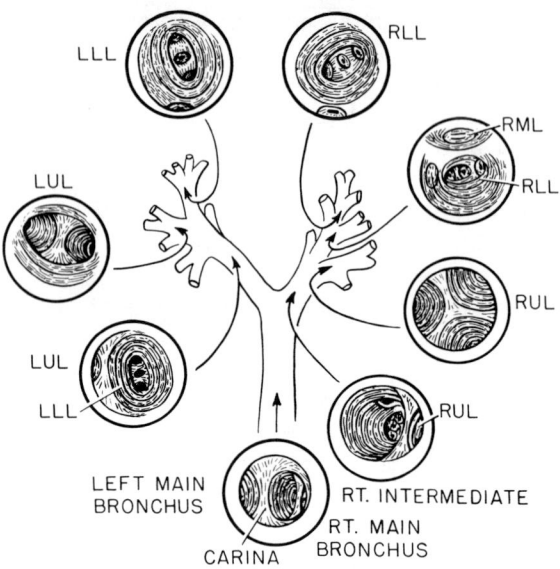

Figure 5.6.
Bronchoscopic view of the various bronchi and their orifices.

Fiberoptic Bronchoscopy

The recent development of the flexible fiberoptic bronchoscope has brought to the bedside an instrument of significant diagnostic as well as therapeutic potential. Clear advantages over the rigid bronchoscope include markedly increased visual range, decreased discomfort for the patient, biopsy of previously inaccessible tumors, and detection of early lung cancer. Biopsies and washings obtained through this instrument may provide critical bacteriologic, histologic, and immunologic information. Because of its larger bore, the older rigid bronchoscope will remain the instrument of choice in the management of major hemoptysis and probably for most extractions of foreign bodies. Basic management skills with this older instrument are, therefore, still necessary. However, for almost all other indications, the flexible fiberoptic bronchoscope can be expected largely to replace it over the next decade. Although its easy portability makes it proper to think of the instrument in its bedside applications, a properly equipped endoscopy suite will improve the diagnostic yield of its use in many cases, particularly in the diagnosis of bronchogenic carcinoma. Fluoroscopic control is frequently required for proper placement of transbronchial biopsy instruments when the tumor is not visible endoscopically.

Fiberoptic bronchoscopy involving biopsy is contraindicated for patients who have uncorrected or uncorrectable bleeding diatheses, and in all cases for those who are uncooperative, who have obstructing tracheal lesions, or who are suffering from active, untreated pulmonary tuberculosis. Prebronchoscopic evaluations, therefore, must include documentation of clotting parameters and cardiovascular function as well as overall respiratory status. In this last category, patients should have, in addition to standard chest x-rays and tomograms for localized disease, pulmonary function studies and arterial blood gas tests. Patients with diminished pulmonary reserve should be considered on an individual basis for this procedure. Although supplemental oxygen may be given during the procedure via either nasal cannulae or tracheal tube adapter, or both, a drop in the patient's Pa_{O_2} of 10 to 20 torr during the procedure is not uncommon. For individuals with a resting room air Pa_{O_2} of below 70 torr, the use of supplemental oxygen before, during, and after the procedure (via nasal prong cannulae) is a wise precaution. The ability to deliver oxygen during fiberoptic bronchoscopy is less than with the rigid bronchoscope and its built-in oxygen cannula. Marked degrees of resting-level hypoxemia or hypercapnea may increase the risk of the procedure beyond its diagnostic or therapeutic potential. Reversible impediments of pulmonary function, such as asthma, bronchitis, or pneumonia, should be corrected if possible before bronchoscopy, and reversible bleeding diatheses should be first improved as well with platelet transfusions, vitamin K, etc. Excessive premedication, which by itself can produce significant hypoxemia, should be avoided in patients with compromised pulmonary reserve, and these high-risk individuals are best monitored on an electrocardiograph during the procedure, for signs of cardiac anoxia.

MATERIAL

Several models of the flexible fiberoptic bronchoscope are currently available on the market (Olympus, American Cystoscope). While differences exist between the models, basically each consists of a flexible shaft carrying three components: the fiberoptic light source, the viewing lens, and a hollow passageway through which lavage and suction are instituted and biopsy instruments passed. The outer diameter of the Olympus BF-B2 model pictured in Figure 5.7 is slightly over 5 mm. Although the techniques to be described are clean and not sterile, the instrument and its biopsy forceps should be carefully sterilized after each case. A defogging solution is applied to the viewing port of the inserted end immediately prior to use.

The remaining material required for the procedure is the same as described above, including the Jackson bronchoscopy kit. Should unexpectedly brisk hemorrhage occur

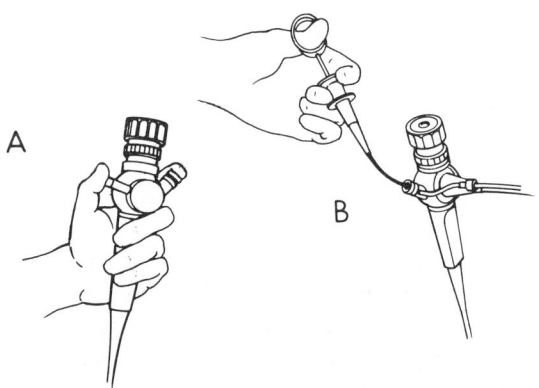

Figure 5.7.

Olympus BF-B2 fiberoptic bronchoscope. (**A**) Demonstrating proper cradling position of the left hand for general viewing purposes. (**B**) With biopsy instrument in place, again showing the correct method of manipulating this attachment.

following biopsy, the small lumen of the fiberoscope biopsy channel will be inadequate to clear it. Therefore, the bronchoscopist must be familiar with and capable of using the Jackson bronchoscope in this emergency situation. As mentioned above, supplemental oxygen should be available to be delivered via nasal cannulae, or the bronchoscope itself may be introduced through a hole cut in a standard oxygen face mask. With high risk patients, electrocardiographic monitoring is valuable. Resuscitation equipment should be at hand.

TECHNIQUE

As with many new procedures, no standard technique has yet evolved for fiberoptic bronchoscopy. Two alternate techniques for insertion of the bronchoscope will be discussed, with the advantages and disadvantages of each pointed out. The procedure should be discussed carefully with the patient in advance, so that he may be prepared for some of the unpleasant sensations he will encounter during bronchoscopy: inability to phonate, coughing and gagging, and a feeling of being unable to get his breath. These should be explained as a direct result of the instrumentation itself, and not dangerous to the patient. An assistant is extremely useful, both in the passage of biopsy forceps and in helping to calm and control the patient during the procedure.

Bronchoscopy Without an Endotracheal Tube

As mentioned above, excessive preparative medication is to be avoided. Atropine 0.4-0.8 mg, plus morphine 5-10 mg or its equivalent, is given intramuscularly 30 minutes before bronchoscopy. If more sedation is desired, hydroxyzine pamoate (Vistaril) 25-50 mg, with its property of lowering airway resistance, is preferred over diazepam (Valium) or the phenothiazines. The patient may be either seated in bed looking straight forward, with the back of the bed up about 60 degrees and the head height at a comfortable level for the examiner, or the procedure may be done with the patient supine. The bronchoscopist and his assistant wear gloves, gowns, and masks. The nasopharynx is examined prior to beginning bronchoscopy. Topical anesthesia of the nasal passageway is induced using direct application of 5 to 10 ml of a 4% solution of cocaine. Viscous Xylocaine is used to lubricate the shaft of the flexible bronchoscope. The tips of the newer instruments will flex 90 degrees in either direction, but older bronchoscopes may flex in only one direction, usually indicated by an arrow on the control knob. The bronchoscopist should check the position of the bronchoscope with regard to its flexing direction and pass it in such a manner that flexing the unit will give him maximum benefit for the particular lesion viewed, without the necessity for rotation. Immediately prior to passage of the scope, Cetacaine spray is used to anesthetize the posterior pharynx. Direct applications of cotton balls soaked in 4% Xylocaine, applied to each pyriform sinus, will reduce gagging. The cross-action laryngeal forceps are used for this procedure. The bronchoscope is passed through the nose, and as it descends the posterior pharynx, the patient is requested to say "e-e-e-e-e." This will approximate the vocal cords, which under direct visualization are lavaged sparingly with 4% Xylocaine, delivered via the irrigating channel of the bronchoscope. The assistant can be extremely useful at this point, injecting the anesthetic through the instrument while the bronchoscopist holds the correct position. After a short wait and relaxation of the cords, an additional 2 to 3 ml of 4% Xylocaine is injected down the trachea. Additional installations of 2% Xylocaine anesthetic solution are used during the case to suppress coughing. The total amount of Xylocaine need rarely exceed 250 mg, and the doses delivered should be monitored scrupulously. Passing the bronchoscope through a curved no. 32 French nasal cannula, placed through the nose after initial application of the topical anesthetic, may ease correct positioning above the vocal cords. Once the vocal cords and tracheobronchial tree are anesthetized, the tube is advanced through the cords (this occasionally requires twisting of the instrument), and visualization of the tracheobronchial tree proceeds in an orderly sequence. Because of the small size of the instrument, all subsegmental orifices should be visualized and entered.

A word should be said here about the preparation for specimens obtained at bronchoscopy. Biopsy bottles, culture tubes, and disposable Luken's tubes (such as the unit incorporating a three-way stopcock manufactured by Rodel) should be at hand and ready for use, with adequate amounts of sterile saline solution (without preservative if cultures are to be taken), drawn up in various syringes for irrigations and washings. The cytotechnician responsible for reading the brushing specimens is consulted in advance regarding the technique he desires for fixing samples. In addition, the pathology department will advise the bronchoscopist regarding initial preparation for special stains, such as the Giemsa or Grocott stains for pneumocystis carinii.

Visible lesions are first brushed directly using the special bristle tip. These minute specimens are freed from the brush and are fixed. The brush may also be washed free in a sterile solution which is then centrifuged, and the sediment is both inoculated on a suitable bacteriologic medium and used for cell block. Prior to concluding the procedure, washings are taken from biopsy sites with the lavage solution introduced via the inner channel and collected into suction by the same route. Biopsy forceps can also be passed via the inner cannula for larger specimens or for transbronchial biopsies. The latter procedure, best performed under fluoroscopy, is a useful diagnostic technique for diagnostically puzzling diffuse diseases of the lung. A small peripheral bronchus in the lower segment is visualized and the forceps is engaged in it. If the patient experiences no chest pain, the forceps is opened on inhalation, closed at the end of exhalation, and slowly retracted. The pulling of lung tissue can be felt and is seen on a fluoroscopic monitor. Three to five biopsies can be obtained in this manner, and in localized disease the forceps can be passed to the lung nodule or density, retracted 0.5 to 1 cm, opened, and then readvanced until resistance is encountered or contact is viewed fluoroscopically. The jaws are then closed and retracted. A special sheathed brush is also available for obtaining anaerobic cultures. The brush is drawn into the sheath before the unit is removed and exposed to atmospheric oxygen. Postbronchoscopic cough specimens are especially valuable and should be collected for the first 24 hours after the procedure. Bleeding should be expected after biopsy, which for this reason is best deferred until the end of the procedure. If brisk bleeding is encountered, the bronchoscope may rapidly become plugged and the bronchoscopist should be prepared to pass a Jackson bronchoscope. Should the patient become short of breath during the procedure, it is best to halt manipulations and allow him to breathe quietly until comfortable. Before the patient is allowed to resume oral intake, the bronchoscopist should return and make sure that his gag reflex has recovered.

The main complication of this procedure, bleeding, is rarely major. The risk of serious hemoptysis is increased by the use of the biopsy forceps, particularly in the transbronchial biopsy of obscure lung lesions in immunosuppressed patients. Pneumothorax is a rare complication, but fever and transient pneumonic infiltrates are occasionally seen, and bronchoscopy should be followed by chest films within 24 hours, particularly if biopsies are taken.

Bronchoscopy With an Endotracheal Tube

In this technique anesthesia is induced in the same manner but without the nasal application of cocaine. With the patient in a sitting position, an 8.5-mm oral endotracheal tube of the flexible, Rusch type, cuffed but not inflated, is slipped over the shaft of the bronchoscope, which is then inserted through the mouth into the tracheobronchial tree, and the endotracheal tube is then advanced over it through the vocal cords. Application of viscous Xylocaine to the distal end of the bronchoscope facilitates passage. As an alternate method, an endotracheal tube with a stylet in the shape indicated in Figure 5.8 may also be inserted into the anesthetized oropharynx over the back of the tongue and epiglottis, in the midline. The position is checked with a finger. When the end of the tube is positioned over the vocal cords the stylet is withdrawn while the tube is pushed forward. The shape of the stylet will cause the distal end of the tube to arc anteriorly and enter the trachea. Five ml of

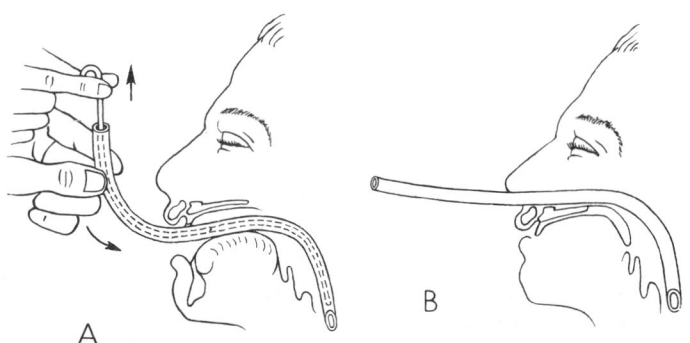

Figure 5.8.

(**A**) Fiberoptic bronchoscopy, demonstrating passage of an endotracheal tube prior to bronchoscopy. A malleable wire stylet is bent as indicated. As the wire is withdrawn, it will cause the tip of the rubber tube to arc forward, allowing this end to be passed forward with the left hand through the larynx. (**B**) Prebronchoscopic nasal tube passage. In this instance the tube is allowed to halt at the level of the epiglottis and is used only as a guide to allow subsequent passage of the fiberoptic bronchoscope into a position above the vocal cords.

2% Xylocaine is injected through the tube into the trachea and the patient is placed supine for passage of the bronchoscope. The advantage of the endotracheal tube is that the bronchoscope can be easily withdrawn, cleaned, and reinserted if the view becomes clouded, or it can be removed to avoid the necessity for withdrawing the biopsy brush the full length of the instrument and thus potentially losing specimens in the biopsy channel. Finally, the endotracheal tube can be used to intubate the opposite lung if postbiopsy bleeding occurs.

The bronchoscope can also be passed through a tracheostomy tube, frequently a particularly valuable maneuver in the management of lobar collapse or persistent atelectasis. It can even be used with a swivel adapter (Portex) that fits into the tracheostomy tube and allows the patient to continue to be ventilated during bronchoscopy. The tracheostomy tube must be larger than 7 mm, and the bronchoscope can cause some leak. To monitor this and to assure adequate alveolar ventilation during the procedure, a spirometer should be attached to the expiratory port of the ventilator.

5.3. PROCTOSIGMOIDOSCOPY

The importance of this examination and of dexterity with the sigmoidoscope is difficult to overemphasize. Digital and anoscopic examinations, plus barium studies, still leave a poorly delineated portion of rectum and lower sigmoid colon that is directly observable through the sigmoidoscope. Of all colonic cancers, 75 percent may be thus visualized, as well as the great majority of inflammatory lesions affecting the colon. The surgeon and physician are therefore equally in need of the information available through its use, and both should make it a routine part of the physical examination in adult patients known to be under increased risk of colonic disease, and certainly as a part of the follow-up of patients with previous colonic disease.

Patients with acute abdominal emergencies may leave the physician little time to prepare the colon prior to inspection, but this circumstance should not prevent the use of the sigmoidoscope in the evaluation of large bowel obstruction or bleeding. Unless mechanical obstruction is suspected, and oral cathartics are therefore contraindicated, the physician will greatly increase the ease and yield of sigmoidoscopy by a previous cleansing of the bowel. Strong, irritative oral cathartics may alter the appearance of the mucosa and are not generally necessary unless barium studies are also planned. Tap water or soapsuds enemas, although effective and sometimes necessary for rapid evacuation, should not be used if possible less than two or three hours prior to the examination, to prevent retained fluid from being a constant annoyance during sigmoidoscopy. A standard and highly successful "dry" preparation consists of three to four Dulcolax tablets the afternoon prior to the day of examination, a liquid and toast supper, and a Dulcolax suppository approximately 3 hours before beginning.

Whenever possible, barium studies should follow rather than precede sigmoidoscopy.

When the luxury of a 24-hour preparative period is inexpedient, or when a barium enema will not be performed, the use of the Dulcolax suppository alone, or a small prepackaged enema, such as the Fleet or Rectalad, two hours before examination, is usually adequate. The enemas again may cause some irritation of the rectal mucosa. In cases of massive rectal bleeding, diarrhea, or inflammatory diseases of the colon, cathartics or enemas are usually not required in any form.

MATERIAL

Sigmoidoscope with obturator and light source, air inflation pump and tubing, cotton swabs on long-handled applicators, biopsy forceps, biopsy jars containing 10% formalin, cautery tip and power source, lubricant, gloves, long suction tip with a suitable aspirating pump.
Comment. Plastic, disposable sigmoidoscopes are now widely available and generally satisfactory. Check the lighting before starting.

TECHNIQUE

The patient will have natural anxieties about this procedure, and these can be allayed considerably, and his cooperation increased—in itself an important asset—by briefly explaining to him before commencing the nature and safety of the examination, as well as the possibility of some discomfort.

Although the head-down position allows the pelvic contents to fall away from the pelvis, and is unquestionably a superior one (Figure 5.9A), it requires the availability of a special examining table not always found on the ward. It may be mimicked in bed or on a low, flat table by the knee-chest position (Figure 5.9B), but it should be remembered that this is an uncomfortable posture after a short time and is poorly tolerated by the elderly. A more leisurely and fully adequate visualization may usually be accomplished by the experienced individual when the patient is in the Sims's or left lateral prone position (Figure 5.9C). Be certain that the patient's buttocks are well out over the edge

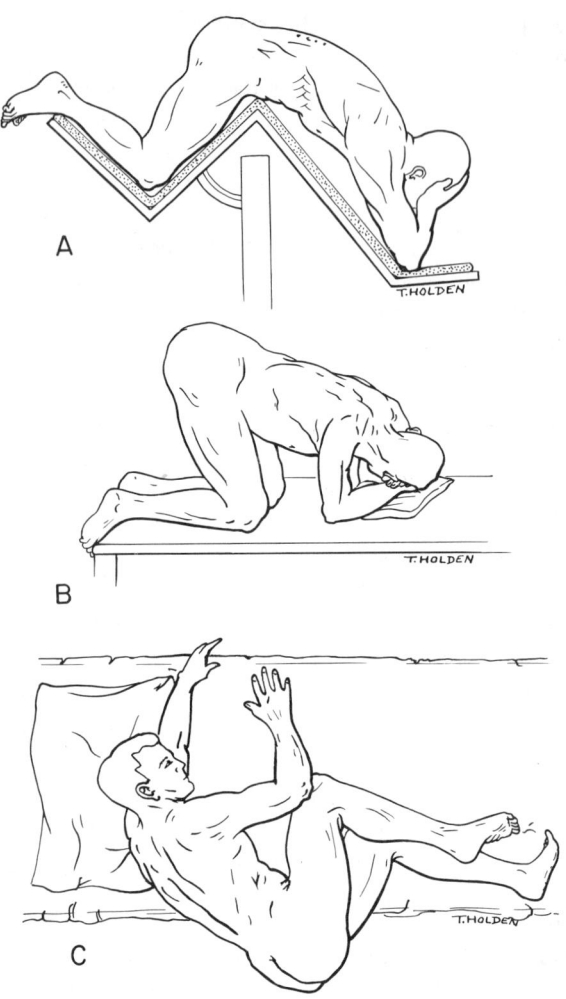

Figure 5.9.

Three common positions for sigmoidoscopy. The usual draping sheets are omitted for clarity. (**A**) Head-down position. (**B**) Knee-chest position. (**C**) Left lateral prone or Sims's position. Note that the buttocks are well out over the edge of the bed.

of the bed or table, and sit in a chair if the height is uncomfortable.

A thorough digital examination of the rectum must precede introduction of the sigmoidoscope. This type of examination not only yields potentially critical information about obstructing or stenotic lesions in the lower rectum, but it also will serve as a mild dilatation of the anus, and, if gently done, will help to ease the patient's mind about what is to follow.

If there is no obstruction or fecal matter in the rectum, proceed with the sigmoidoscopy. Run warm water over the metal obturator to reduce the discomfort of cold steel on bare skin, then lubricate the instrument generously for its full length. Attach the inflation bag. Inform the patient before inserting the tip and ask him to bear down slightly, thus dilating the anal sphincters. Separate the buttocks with the thumb and forefinger of the left hand, and introduce the tip of the sigmoidoscope gently and slowly for a distance of 3 or 4 cm, in the general direction of the umbilicus, until the tip is past the bulge of the prostate in the male or of the cervix in the female. If the obturator is the long-handled type, hold it in place with the thumb of the right hand during introduction. Remove the obturator and attach the light source.

There are obviously two periods during sigmoidoscopy when bowel visualization is possible: during advancement of the instrument and during its withdrawal. Inspection should be leisurely and complete; therefore, it follows that the most careful observations should be made when the patient is experiencing least discomfort, i.e., during withdrawal. Lesions seen during entry should be noted, of course, but the prime responsibility is to do a complete examination, and this requires full-length passage of the sigmoidoscope, as rapidly and painlessly as feasible. In addition, biopsies performed during entry may result in bleeding that renders full examination impossible. Spontaneous bleeding points are best appreciated during introduction, however, because those first seen at a later time may be secondary to trauma.

Follow the lumen of the bowel, using inflation sparingly

and only when the lumen is not discernible. In disease states such as ulcerative colitis, in which the bowel is notoriously fragile, air insufflation is best avoided altogether if possible, and the danger of perforation may preclude full advancement. An invisible lumen may become clear simply by pushing aside the eyepiece and allowing retained gas to escape, thus collapsing and telescoping the bowel about the tube. Other guides to the correct path are fluid streams from higher levels, bubbles, or fecal contents. Should the rectum contain large quantities of feces, the preparation has been inadequate, and both patient and examiner will be spared needless frustration by desisting at once and returning after a proper evacuation has been obtained.

Under no circumstances should force be used to advance the sigmoidoscope. This is the single most common method of producing a rent even in normal bowel. If the patient is in the knee-chest position, deep breathing through the mouth will relax his abdominal musculature and also allow the pelvic contents to fall forward.

The rectum rapidly curves into the sacral hollow as it ascends, and following it will require the sigmoidoscope to be directed posteriorly and then the examiner's head to be dropped toward the bed when using the knee-chest position, or sideways toward the bed if the patient is in the Sims position (having the patient's buttocks well out over the edge of the bed allows room to perform this maneuver gracefully). The inferior valve of Houston may be seen in this area on the left posterior wall. Advance the sigmoidoscope gently, holding it between the thumb and forefinger of the dominant hand. As the rectum next comes forward over the sacral promontory, the end of the instrument usually will describe an arc of about 60 degrees away from the bed, and the middle valve of Houston should become visible on the right anterior wall. The superior valve lies also on the right anterior wall about 13 cm from the anus, and 2 or 3 cm further, the rectum angulates sharply into the sigmoid colon, usually to the patient's left, but occasionally to the right. This corner may well be a 90-degree bend, and traversing it is the most difficult portion of the examination, particularly in those patients unable to flex their spines because of degenerative changes. The judicious use of air insufflation plus repeated withdrawals and advances will often ease the passage.

Once the sigmoidoscope has been inserted its full 25 cm, withdrawal should be slow and should allow 360-degree visualization at all times. Remember the ampullary nature of the terminal rectum and check the blind area directly posterior to the sphincters before final removal; also examine the dentate line and its vicinity at this time.

Biopsy
Small polyps may be removed with a loop snare or biopsy forceps, and the base cauterized after aspiration of the potentially inflammable colonic gas. Larger and sessile lesions may have punch biopsies removed for diagnostic studies, but complete excision is better reserved for the operating room, with blood available. Cauterization should be thorough, for bleeding can be active enough to render a second effort impossible. Extreme caution should be taken to avoid overly deep biopsies, particularly of shallow inflammatory ulcers, or of any lesion on the thin anterior rectal wall; deep biopsies are not necessary, and they can be dangerous. Bowel perforation above the peritoneal reflection (over 10 cm from the anal opening) often requires colostomy diversion, whereas that at a lower level usually drains into the bowel and does not require surgery. Barium studies performed shortly after a biopsy carry the hazard of barium extravasation through a small, unsuspected perforation, or through a weakened area caused by the biopsy. If at all possible, therefore, delay x-rays for 48 hours.

5.4. FIBEROPTIC GASTROSCOPY

The development of the fiberoptic gastroscope has brought the diagnostic use of gastroscopy to the patient's bedside. In contrast to most other bedside techniques described in this book, however, facility with the use of this specialized instrument, as well as judgment in evaluating what is seen through it, must be acquired through prior experience with elective gastroscopies. In general, bedside gastroscopy is indicated for a single problem: acute upper gastrointestinal hemorrhage. Although the role of the fiberoptic gastroscope in diagnosing sites of origin for upper intestinal bleeding is still developing, certain guidelines in logistics have emerged. Bedside gastroscopy should be considered in patients whose vital signs are reasonably stable, but whose overall condition or monitoring equipment make transportation to an endoscopy suite impractical. Gastroscopy should be performed before barium studies.

MATERIAL

Different models of fiberoptic gastroscopes are available, but each incorporates certain controls in common, and the operator should be thoroughly familiar with them in advance and should have an experienced gastroscopist with him if he has not attempted this procedure before. The endoscope has controls for the introduction of air and water as well as a suction channel for clearing gastric contents and removing clots from the surface of lesions in the stomach. For diagnostic studies in the patient with acute upper gastrointestinal hemorrhage, the endviewing panendoscope is the most useful optical configuration. Floor supplies: Cetacaine or other topical anesthetic, 0.5% Pontocaine, cross-action laryngeal forceps, cotton pledgets, Ewalt tube.

TECHNIQUE

Two criteria must be met before a patient can be considered as a candidate for bedside gastroscopy. An Ewalt tube, passed immediately prior to gastroscopy in an attempt to empty the stomach, must be able to clear the gastric cavity of fresh blood. Lavage contents should be returned clear or suggestive of old clots. If bleeding continues at a rate that cannot be cleared by an Ewalt tube, adequate visualization of the gastric wall will be impossible; however, the esophagus can be viewed, even in the massively bleeding individual. Also, when the Ewalt tube is passed, some judgment can be made about the patient's degree of cooperation. Whereas

5 to 15 mg of Valium, given slowly intravenously, is suggested in patients whose vital signs are stable, as a sedative prior to fiberoptic gastroscopy, the retching, gagging patient will destroy the calm atmosphere necessary for a thorough examination.

The procedure is discussed with the patient and explained in detail. The patient should be made to understand that some retching is not unusual and that this can often be managed by breathing deeply, or panting like a dog. He should also be instructed to resist urges to swallow on the tube itself. The Ewalt tube will have given him the sensation of the gastroscope in advance. Prior to passing the gastroscope, however, the posterior pharynx is anesthetized with a surface active agent such as Cetacaine in a spray bottle, and the valecullae are swabbed with cotton pledgets, soaked in 0.5% Pontocaine or 4% Xylocaine, on cross-action laryngeal forceps. Whenever possible, two individuals should be present, as well as a nurse to comfort the patient. One individual passes the gastroscope in its initial course while the other views.

The patient is placed flat on his left side with head flexed slightly forward. The distal end of the unit is held between the fingers like a pencil, and the instrument is then fed into the posterior pharynx through the open mouth. The index finger guides it into the esophagus while the viewer can see the epiglottis as it is passed and assists in proper direction. The esophagus is observed for bleeding varices or other lesions, and the stomach is entered. In general, air is used to distend the stomach while water is used to clear the end of the gastroscope of clots or food particles, and suction is employed to clear away blood or infused water. After the gastroscope passes the gastroesophageal junction, the stomach is distended with air. The gastroscope is now bent via its controls to a right angle position, and by rotating it on its long axis the entire contents of the stomach are visible, except for those areas in the immediate vicinity of the gastroesophageal junction. The gastroscope is advanced until it rests against the pylorus, which will usually open with slight pressure and allow the tip of the instrument to advance into the duodenum. To view finally the area of the stomach high on the lesser curvature near the esophagus, or in the fundic portion of the stomach, a maneuver called retroflexion is performed. The end of the gastroscope is pulled back into the stomach and is curved against the pylorus in such a manner that it turns back on itself. The success of this maneuver is indicated when the proximal portion of the gastroscope itself is visible to the viewer. The end of the panendoscope is now pointing toward the gastro-esophageal junction, and these areas around it may be visualized. Fundic bleeding sites are notoriously difficult to locate, but with persistence this area can usually be brought into focus.

6.

RESPIRATORY TECHNIQUES

6.1. NASAL OXYGEN CATHETERS

The simple placement of a nasal oxygen catheter is a prime example of the importance of detail. Should the catheter be inserted far enough to allow it to curve downward in the posterior pharynx, a dangerous degree of gastric insufflation and abdominal distension can follow. This is particularly likely to occur in the unconscious or heavily sedated patient. A 4-cm to 5-cm penetration is fully adequate in most people, but a rough estimate of the distance from the nares to the posterior border of the soft palate can be made in each individual by holding the catheter next to the face (Figure 6.1) before inserting it. Once in place, the pharynx should be inspected, and if the catheter is visible, it should be withdrawn the proper distance.

The routine use of nasal oxygen catheters in the postoperative patient is ill advised. Correctly placed catheters can still result in varying degrees of air swallowing and distension during the phase of recovery from anesthesia, and the humidification of the gas stream is not usually sufficient to prevent some drying and irritation of the nasopharyngeal mucosa. Evaluate each patient for need, *and remove these catheters as soon as the need is past.*

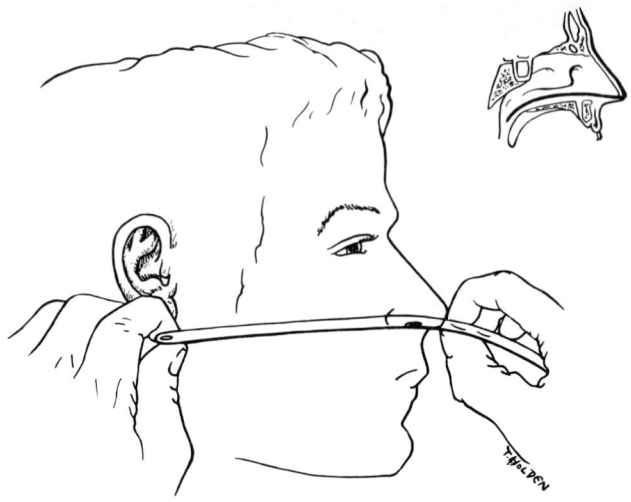

Figure 6.1.

Proper length for insertion of a nasal catheter may usually be estimated by marking off on the tube a length equal to the distance from the tip of the nose to the tragus of the ear.

6.2. ENDOTRACHEAL SUCTION

Mechanical cleansing of the trachea by catheter suction is indicated whenever the patient is unable to clear his own secretions. With the prevalence of chronic lung disease in our population, it is not surprising to find such conditions arising with equal frequency on the medical and surgical services. They include overwhelming pneumonia, cerebrovascular accidents, postoperative patients with painful abdominal or thoracic incisions, and practically any illness in the severely debilitated. The frequent use of nasal oxygen with its drying tendency, the loss of respiratory stimulus secondary to this oxygen, and the use of narcotic analgesics make coughing and deep breathing exercises an essential part of the preparation for surgery in the elderly.

Nevertheless, despite the most diligent preoperative efforts and continued use of every respiratory aid postoperatively, the physician will be faced almost daily with this typical individual: somnolent, with a feeble cough and audible tracheal secretions, febrile, with poor breath sounds at the bases of his lungs, and with areas of atelectasis or frank pneumonia on chest film. For such a patient, endotracheal suction offers two great aids. (1) It will mechanically remove some of the obstructing, often purulent secretions; and (2) of equal importance, the patient will, unless moribund, be stimulated to a vigorous and productive period of coughing.

The technique by its nature is an extremely uncomfortable one for the patient, who will come to fear deep suctioning with an almost religious intensity. Despite this, it should be employed as often as required, and the very possibility of its recurrence can often coax a cough from the most recalcitrant. Remember that endotracheal suctioning is not always adequate, and it is not without hazard.

MATERIAL

Sterile gloves, water-soluble lubricant, dry sponges, sterile suction catheter, nos. 12 or 14 French red rubber catheter connected by a glass or plastic T-tube adapter to a suction line, Gomco, or other pump suction device if wall suction is unavailable, culture swabs and tubes, saline solution-filled 20-ml syringe, and oxygen line which can be fitted to the T-tube adapter in place of the suction line.

Comment. The Bard-Parker prepackaged no. 14 plastic Reguvac suction catheter (Figure 6.2) is also excellent. The T-tube is an integral section of the tube, the additional stiffness of the plastic is useful, and the tips are open-ended.

TECHNIQUE

An assistant is essential. The patient is sitting in bed, close to upright, with the shoulders supported, but no pillow behind the head or neck. If supplemental oxygen is being used, it should be continued until the moment of intubation. Stand on the patient's right side if right-handed, vice versa if left-handed, while the assistant stands on the opposite side of the bed. Although the suction catheter will pass through the patient's nose and oropharynx, wear gloves to prevent additional contamination. Lubricate the catheter and connect it to the suction source, but vent it through the T-tube

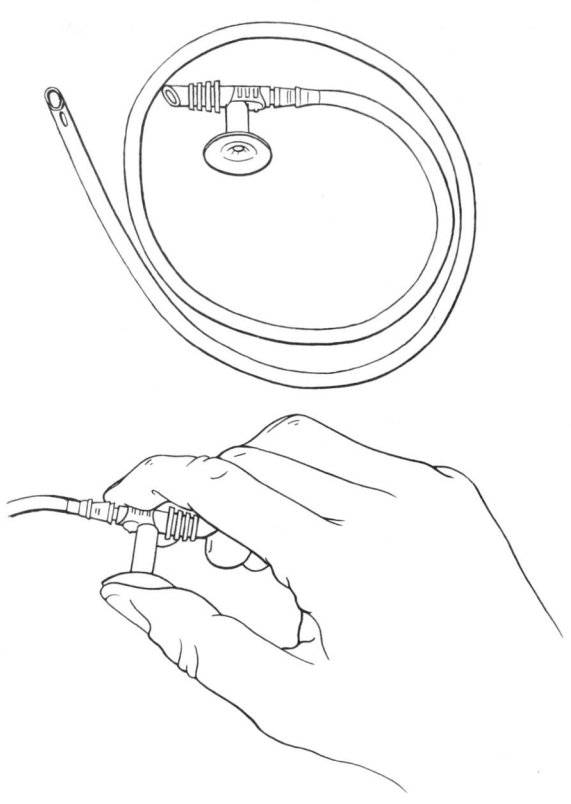

Figure 6.2.

Reguvac endotracheal suction catheter. Suction control is integral part of unit.

and do not apply negative pressure until actually within the trachea. Endotracheal suctioning will be a frightening sensation for the patient, who should be instructed in the nature of the procedure, told that he or she will be forced to cough, and will be unable to speak when the catheter is in place.

If the assistant now grasps the tongue with the dry sponge and pulls it forward gently in the midline, it will, in turn, pull the epiglottis anteriorly and leave the trachea more accessible. Some operators prefer to reserve this maneuver until other efforts have failed. Pass the catheter straight back along the floor of the nasal passageway and allow it to curve downward in the pharynx. Do not hesitate to change nares if there is obstruction, and do not use suction as the catheter advances.

The tip of the tube can usually be felt to strike the resistance of the epiglottis even when it is pulled forward. At this point, instruct the patient to cough or to say "e-e-e-e-e" in a high-pitched voice, and as he phonates and pushes the epiglottis further forward, rapidly advance the tip into the trachea. Successful intubation will be heralded by strong coughing, loss of voice, and a characteristically hollow quality of breathing. It is at this point that suctioning begins.

During the actual suctioning process, blood oxygenation has been shown to plummet sharply, and strong vagal stimuli are elicited. In the enfeebled patient who needs endotracheal suctioning, unwisely prolonged application of it has caused cardiac arrest. A sharp alertness for the patient's adequate oxygenation should therefore be uppermost. One helpful reminder is for the physician to hold his own breath while suctioning, releasing the T-tube as soon as he feels a desire to breathe again, and applying an oxygen catheter in place of the suction tubing to restore blood aeration. Swabs from the T-tube may be sent for cultures during this period. With suction off and the catheter not actually moving in the trachea, the patient will usually stop coughing and breathe easier. Thus, by judicious use of intermittent periods of rest, the catheter may be left in place longer and achieve better results. Saline solution or diluted mucolytic agents such as Alevaire may be directly instilled into the trachea through the tube in 5-ml to 10-ml aliquots to aid further in dissolution of mucous plugs. Turning the head to one side will favor passage of the catheter tip into the opposite mainstem bronchus, and differential cleansing is often possible. Two to three minutes in the trachea are adequate to accomplish the goal; further stimulation will usually yield little, but will exhaust the patient.

Because of the potential dangers, endotracheal suctioning

should be done only by a doctor or a specifically trained assistant, with oxygen and resuscitation equipment available. Pharyngeal and deep pharyngeal suctioning, accomplished in the same manner but without entering the trachea, is often carried out by nurses on the wards and intensive care units. The coughing and gagging attendant upon even this type of aspiration can also produce the same serious drop in blood oxygen levels. If tragic accidents are to be avoided, *all personnel who perform this service must be fully aware of its hazards and must be warned specifically of the dangers of prolonged suctioning.*

As described, tracheal intubation appears technically simple, yet in many patients it is not, because of either local anatomy or an active gag reflex. Turning the head from side to side, leaning the patient forward, or even trying the approach through the opposite nostril may help, but gentleness with the catheter tip is most important. Success is not always possible, and in these cases efforts should not persist unduly; even deep pharyngeal suctioning will often produce effective coughing.

The availability of ultrasonic nebulizers has greatly increased the penetrating and mucolytic effectiveness of water vapor. The intermittent use of these machines can sharply augment the productiveness of endotracheal suction.

6.3. TRANSTRACHEAL COUGH CATHETER

A useful technique with those patients in whom endotracheal suctioning is difficult or unduly hazardous is the use of the transtracheal cough catheter. Although obviously lacking the advantage of mechanical cleansing, its use will stimulate productive coughing, and its presence is well tolerated. Mucolytic agents such as Alevaire and Mucomyst may be used through such a catheter in addition to saline solution.

The development of subcutaneous emphysema is a reported complication of this technique, but this problem is very infrequent, can usually be avoided by use of a small catheter, and does not, at any rate, outweigh the usefulness of the procedure. The catheter does represent a potential pathway for pulmonary infection, and it should be maintained as sterile as possible—48 to 72 hours is a reasonable time limit to set for such a cannula, although cannulas of this type have been left in place for considerably longer periods of time without apparent ill effect.

MATERIAL

Medium-size Intracath (17-gauge, 2-inch needle), dry and antiseptic-soaked gauze sponges, syringe with no. 25 needle containing local anesthetic, 1-inch tape (torn in several 3-inch strips), syringe containing 5 to 10 ml sterile saline solution.

TECHNIQUE

The patient is in a semisitting position with the neck extended; this position is best accomplished by instructing him to look at the ceiling. The catheter will pass through the center of the cricothyroid membrane, and this area should first be accurately localized. It is most easily found by first locating the peaked superior margin of the thyroid cartilage and then palpating inferiorly until the lower edge of this cartilage is just passed. Inasmuch as the position of the membrane will change with swallowing, the patient should be instructed to resist the urge until the catheter is in place.

After skin preparation a small wheal of local anesthetic is raised in the midline over the cricothyroid membrane. The Intracath is then passed in a single motion through skin, subcutaneous tissue, and membrane, at right angles to each, and with the *bevel of the needle down* (Figure 6.3). Quickly feed about 5 cm of catheter down the trachea and remove the needle carefully. The patient may cough briefly when the needle penetrates the trachea, but the catheter itself will not stimulate him. If the inner sleeve does not pass easily, it means that the trachea has not been entered or that the needle is impinged upon the posterior wall of the trachea. In either case, it is better to withdraw to a superficial location and try again. A small sterile dressing is taped in place

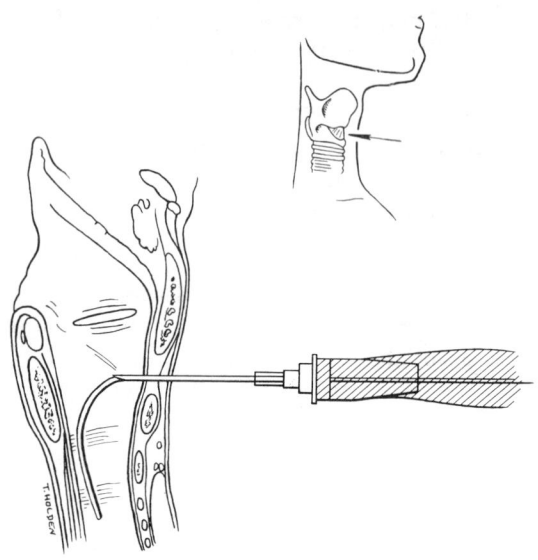

Figure 6.3.

Transtracheal cough catheter. Intracath pierces cricothyroid membrane at right angles. Needle bevel is down.

over the puncture site, and the catheter itself is taped to the neck distal to the needle point as protection in the unlikely event of the needle shearing off the catheter, even though sheathed. The needle is left plugged, but is opened at 2-hour to 3-hour intervals for the administration of 5-ml or 10-ml aliquots of saline or diluted mucolytic solutions. Suction on the syringe, immediately after instillation of saline solution and while the patient is still coughing, will also produce tracheal specimens suitable for culture. Several reports have attested the superiority of this technique in obtaining standard cultures of the respiratory flora.

Although the Intracath is convenient for this technique, the same results may be accomplished by passing a suitable polyethylene catheter through a large-bore needle piercing the cricothyroid membrane. The needle is then removed, a blunt-tipped needle is fitted to the line, and the catheter is used in the same manner. A needle with an obturator is preferable, for the presence of the obturator prevents tissue from clogging the bore and thus blocking subsequent passage of the catheter.

6.4. EMERGENCY TRACHEOSTOMY

Prompt consultation and an early decision usually will eliminate the necessity for a bedside tracheostomy. The superiority of operating-room personnel, lighting, and suction are three compelling reasons for the performance of this procedure in proper surroundings. Occasionally, the immobility of a patient's life-supporting equipment will justify a bedside tracheostomy, but rarely is anyone "too sick" to tolerate a carefully monitored journey to the operating room. Decisive evaluation of upper-airway obstruction, overwhelming pulmonary secretions, repeated aspirations, or inadequate ventilatory effort, *before the patient has weakened to the point of exhaustion and imminent asphyxiation,* can avoid the desperate midnight gamble beside an ill-lit bed, the setting in which the majority of tracheostomy complications occur. In such emergency situations, the passage of an endotracheal tube can still supply the respiratory support required to allow transfer to the operating room. Acute reversible conditions (aspiration, pulmonary edema, cardiac arrest) so treated may never require tracheostomy.

When choosing initially between tracheostomy and endotracheal intubation, the length of time respiratory control will be needed is a critical factor. The ability to aspirate the trachea is less adequate with an endotracheal tube, and heavy sedation is often required. After 48 to 72 hours, these two drawbacks, plus the danger of laryngeal and vocal cord edema, will begin to outweigh the benefits of a return to anatomic normality.

A severe, uncorrected hemorrhagic diathesis is a contraindication to tracheostomy. Pediatric tracheostomies should be performed only by the experienced, and never at the bedside.

MATERIAL

Emergency tracheostomy kit: single-cuffed low-pressure balloon, or double-cuffed tracheostomy tubes (Figure 6.4) in nos. 32, 34, and 36 French sizes, suction catheters and tubing adapters, scalpel handle, curved Metzenbaum scissors, straight suture scissors, 2 pairs of tissue forceps with teeth, 6 curved and 6 straight Halsted hemostatic forceps, 4 Kelly clamps, tracheal hook, 2 U.S. Army pattern retractors, 2 Senn double-ended retractors, 2 Weitlander self-retaining retractors, 2 Allis tissue forceps, 4-0 and 2-0 catgut ligatures, 4-0 silk skin sutures, cloth tape for tracheostomy tube collar, 2 syringes, 25-gauge and 22-gauge needles, ampules of local anesthetic, 2 gowns, 6 towels, 4 towel clips, gauze sponges. Floor supplies: Suction tubing, suction apparatus, culture swabs and tubes, strong bedside or gooseneck lamp, 20-ml syringe with adapter to fit inflation tubing of tracheostomy tube, rubber-shod Kelly clamp for this tubing, sterile gloves, masks, caps, antiseptic solution, adhesive tape.

Comment. Although this assortment of tube sizes is generally adequate, both larger and smaller sizes should be readily available. The balloons must be tested for leaks and uniformity of expansion before beginning. If a plastic tube is to be used, it may be soaked in hot water for 15 minutes, with the balloon inflated, to increase its pliability.

TECHNIQUE

This procedure ideally requires four individuals: operator, assistant, floor nurse, and anesthesiologist or oxygen therapist. If the patient is being converted from controlled respiration via an endotracheal tube to a tracheostomy tube, it is usually desirable to have the anesthesiologist or oxygen therapist detach the respirator and control the patient's breathing during the tracheostomy with a manual unit fitted to the endotracheal tube, such as the Ambu bag. If the patient does not have such a tube in place, an anesthesiologist can assist him with face mask respiration, and can be prepared to pass an endotracheal tube, should he suddenly become obstructed or suffer an arrest during the operation. The nurse should be used to adjust the lighting and help to

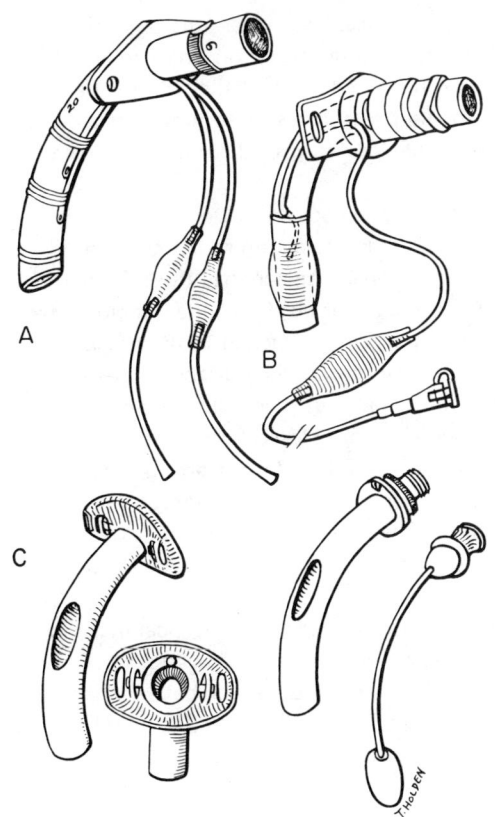

Figure 6.4.

Common types of tracheostomy tubes. (**A**) Double-cuffed red rubber tube. The balloons are alternatively inflated to lessen the danger of tracheal erosion. (**B**) Single-cuffed plastic tube. The low-pressure cuffed tracheostomy tube has a similar appearance, but the balloon is more floppy. (**C**) Fenestrated silver tube with fenestrated inner cannula and olive-tipped introducer. Matching apertures of inner and outer cannulas allow the patient to speak and breathe more normally. Replacing the inner cannula with an unperforated one converts this tube functionally to a standard tracheostomy tube.

restrain the patient if necessary. *Do not attempt a tracheostomy in feeble lighting.*

If the patient is conscious, he will probably be terrified. Sedation is usually contraindicated, but a few words of explanation and encouragement can help to relieve him, and by reducing his struggles, greatly ease the operation. The neck should be fully extended by placing a rolled blanket or pillow behind the shoulders and allowing the head to fall back against the mattress. If respiratory distress is severe, tracheostomy can be performed with the patient in a semi-sitting position.

Gloves, gowns, masks, and caps are worn. The entire anterior surface of the neck, from chin to upper chest, is carefully cleansed and draped. Anesthetize the skin in a vertical midline from the lower border of the cricoid cartilage to the suprasternal notch. A tracheostomy may be accomplished satisfactorily through a horizontal incision, but the following points favor the vertical incision:

1. Because the incision is not closed tightly, and a large tube protrudes from its central portion, scarring is usually equal for both horizontal and vertical incisions.

2. Tracheal secretions will tend to pool behind the lower flap of a horizontal incision, creating the potential for a wound infection.

3. Tracheal exposure is superior via the vertical incision when the neck is short.

Dissection is carried down in the midline between the strap muscles, which are retracted laterally. This line may be recognized as a thin whitish raphe, and may not be in the center of the incision. Frequent palpation of the trachea is the best safeguard against wandering off course. The anterior jugular and inferior thyroid veins will usually be distended, and they should be carefully divided and ligated when necessary. The most common immediate complication of tracheostomy is bleeding. Unless the urgency of establishing an airway is great, meticulous hemostasis should be achieved before the tracheostomy tube is in place, and in the way.

Immediately anterior to the trachea is a layer of fibrofatty tissue that must be divided to expose the tracheal rings, and also the isthmus of the thyroid gland. The problems of cricoid cartilage erosion and laryngeal stricture are associated with tracheostomy tubes placed too high; both the second and third tracheal rings should be transected.

Ordinarily, the thyroid isthmus can be retracted superiorly to allow placement of the tube. If this is not possible, divide the gland between Kelly clamps. Dissection close to the trachea may precipitate violent paroxysms of coughing that can further embarrass the patient's ventilation. If an endotracheal tube is not in place, 2 to 3 ml of 1% Xylocaine, instilled directly into the trachea, will abolish this reflex.

The tip of the tracheal hook is now passed beneath the lower border of the second ring and the trachea is pulled gently anteriorly. (Skim the point of the hook under the cartilage to avoid puncturing the balloon of an endotracheal tube.) Carefully incise the trachea along the upper border of the ring for a distance of 1.5 cm. Grasp the second ring in the Allis forceps, remove the tracheal hook, and maintaining light traction on the trachea, cut inferiorly across either one or two rings at each end of the initial incision, to create a square flap of trachea, hinged at the bottom. There are several methods of handling the tracheostomy aperture; three of the more common ones are illustrated in Figure 6.5. Suturing the flap to the platysma (the stitch to be removed later) allows easy entry into the trachea for bronchoscopy and tube replacement. It also causes necrosis of the tracheal flap. Two sutures of heavy silk, passed through a cartilage ring on either side of the opening, led out of the incision in the neck and tied to form two loops, can be used as handles to pull the trachea up into this incision if the tracheostomy tube should be inadvertently pulled out. Simple excision of the flap is usually adequate.

If the patient is not on endotracheal support, the trachea should be thoroughly aspirated before inserting the tube. If he is, the endotracheal tube is removed immediately prior to insertion of the tracheostomy tube. The largest tube accommodated comfortably by the opening is now introduced and the balloon inflated to secure an airtight seal between tube and tracheal wall. The forcible passage of a tube too large for the tracheostomy may result in a granulation tissue response that can lead to late tracheal stenosis. Attach the tracheostomy tube to the respirator, and tie the tube in place by means of two unequal lengths of cloth tape

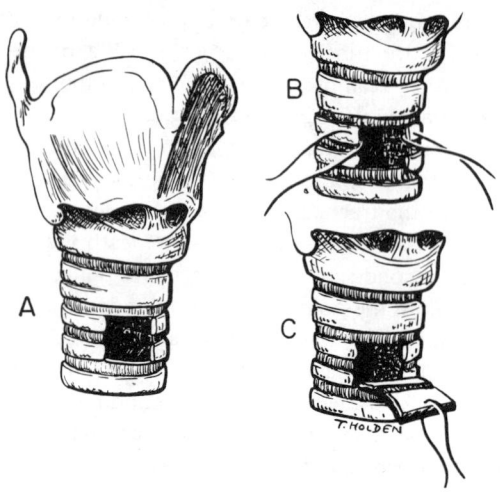

Figure 6.5.

(**A**) Standard tracheostomy aperture. Two rings are cut. (**B**) Sutures through cartilages, along each lateral wall of tracheal aperture, pass free through the open incision and may be used to pull trachea forward. (**C**) Tracheal flap is sutured to subcutaneous tissue.

(so that the knot will be visible on the side of the neck), passed through the openings in the tube flange and tied snugly about the neck. *These tapes must be tight;* the inflated cuff itself will not prevent dislodgment of the tube during coughing or turning.

A full closure of the tracheostomy incision is unwise. It not only favors the formation of subcutaneous emphysema, but more importantly, it also blocks the egress of tracheal secretions, thus setting up the potential for a wound infection. A few stitches may be placed at either corner of the incision, or it may be left completely open. A 4 × 4 gauze dressing, slit in the center, is fitted around the tube and under the tapes. Before leaving the patient, auscultate both lungs carefully for adequate ventilation. The tube may have entered a main stem bronchus, cutting off the flow of air to the opposite lung. Massive atelectasis and collapse will occur rapidly unless the balloon is deflated and the tube is withdrawn slowly until breath sounds are heard over both lungs. Decreased breath sounds and hyperresonance to percussion should also alert the surgeon to the possibility of a pneumothorax. This complication is not uncommon following a stormy bedside tracheostomy and is presumably caused by puncturing the cupola of the pleura in the neck or by dissection of air into the mediastinum and subsequent rupture of the mediastinal pleura. Because a small pneumothorax can enlarge rapidly under positive pressure ventilation, a postoperative chest x-ray is prudent, and a high degree of suspicion should be maintained if the patient's aeration is less than expected.

Tracheostomy Care

Tracheostomy care is an exacting and time-consuming task. However, competence in the management of these patients must be developed if the common complications of this operation are to be avoided. Although the immediate problems secondary to the surgery have been mentioned in the Technique section, later difficulties usually group themselves in the following three interrelated categories.

Airway Obstruction
A nurse must be in constant attendance with any patient on assisted ventilation. A malfunctioning respirator is a totally effective garrotte, but it may sound normal. Close observation of respiratory excursions, color, and vital signs is essential. Humidification of the inspired gases, via either a Briggs adapter or a nebulizer on the respirator, reduces drying of secretions and airway blockage and thus makes suctioning more effective and less frequently needed. Overfilling of a nebulizer fed by a continuous drip, however, can drown the patient.

The loss of an effective cough will make suctioning necessary when secretions become audible, or atelectasis occurs because of their retention. *Prolonged suctioning can cause severe hypoxia and cardiac arrest,* but it may be safely repeated if the patient is allowed to become oxygenated through the use of an oxygen catheter in the tracheostomy tube between aspirations. Irrigations with 10 ml of sterile saline solution by a physician can loosen plugs. Ventilatory assistance should not be interrupted for suctioning for more than 15 seconds.

Tracheostomy tubes without inner cannulae are replaced by clean ones 48 to 72 hours after insertion. Because a tract may not yet be well established, this first exchange might be difficult and should be performed by a physician. Inner cannulae of plastic or silver tubes should be removed at 8-hour intervals, cleansed, sterilized, and replaced. Obstructive complications associated with the use of cuffed tubes include displacement of the balloon beyond the end of the tube, rubber tube kinkage, slippage of the tube into a main stem bronchus, and aspiration of pharyngeal or gastric secretions on deflation of the cuff.

Physical therapy by experienced specialists can be of great help in freeing the patient of occluding secretions. If he can tolerate frequent turning onto prone, lateral, and supine positions, with vigorous chest and cough therapy in each position, basilar atelectasis and pneumonitis can often be avoided or successfully treated. While on the respirator, the patient may be "sighed" intermittently, usually by allowing two inflow cycles while blocking the expiratory phase between them. This simulates a deep breath and also helps to prevent atelectasis.

Infection

A tracheostomy opens a direct path between the lungs and the organisms in the outside environment. Aspiration of secretions and tracheal toilet are both important safeguards against excessive colonization of the trachea with pathogens, but they must be accomplished with a standardized, rigidly aseptic technique if inadvertent seeding of bacteria is to be avoided. Disposable, sterile suction catheters are used, and sterile gloves are used in passing them. Aspiration samples for cultures should be taken regularly to alert the physician to changing flora, particularly if antibiotic therapy has been instituted. The cut 4 × 4 gauze square (not cotton filled), is changed frequently to prevent skin irritation and to remove pooled secretions from the incision. The area may be washed with benzalkonium chloride before applying the new dressing. Respiratory machinery tubing should be regularly inspected and cultured, particularly if one piece of equipment has been used continuously for several days without sterilization.

Trauma to the Tracheobronchial Tree

Severe tracheal irritation and bleeding secondary to tracheal suctioning can usually be avoided by first moistening the catheter with sterile saline solution and by being gentle with the tip during aspiration. To reduce the likelihood of pressure necrosis, low-pressure balloon tubes should be employed whenever possible. The cuffs of a double-cuffed tube are alternately deflated every two hours, *after first aspirating the pharynx clear of secretions.* The empty balloon is first inflated, then the full one deflated. Regardless of the type of balloon system employed, fill the cuff with a minimum pressure; 8 to 15 ml of air is just enough to prevent air leak into the mouth during positive pressure ventilation. The requirement for progressively greater amounts of air in the balloon should warn the physician of the possible development of tracheomalacia.

Be prepared to suction the trachea for secretions which may escape as the cuff is deflated.

Single cuffs are also deflated for a few moments every 2 hours after pharyngeal suction.

Removal of the Tracheostomy Tube

Criteria for successful weaning from a tracheostomy tube vary with the disease under treatment, and a full discussion of them is beyond the purposes of this book. Progressively occluding corks with a fenestrated tube may be useful if an underlying chronic pulmonary disorder is present. For fully reversible conditions, this apparatus is often not required.

Serial blood gas determinations, as respiratory assistance and oxygen supplementation are systematically withdrawn, has emerged today as by far the most objective and valuable tool in predicting the feasibility of tube withdrawal.

7.

NASAL PACKING

The majority of nosebleeds are anterior in location and are caused by trauma, including the chronic irritation of nose picking, and rhinitis secondary to upper respiratory infections. Hypertension and arteriosclerosis have also been implicated, as have on occasion such diverse diseases as rheumatic fever and leukemia. Posterior bleeding is rarely due to trauma, but usually represents the splitting of a sclerotic vessel, exacerbated by hypertension. Patients seldom have epistaxis secondary to a clotting defect, however, unless it is of a degree that manifests itself with generalized bleeding into other mucous membranes or skin, and leaves little doubt as to the diagnosis. Inadequate nasal packing, followed by medications to combat a presumed clotting disorder, is a common compound of clinical errors.

MATERIAL
Head mirror, nasal speculum, bayonet forceps, epinephrine in 1:1000 dilution, silver nitrate applicators, 5% cocaine or 2% Pontocaine (tetracaine) hydrochloride, petrolatum-impregnated anterior nasal packing, posterior nasal packs, cotton balls, gauze sponges, red rubber suction catheter, and basin for the patient to hold. A bright bare-bulb light is essential, and a constant-suction apparatus will prove useful.

Comment. Anterior packing in the proper narrow widths is available in foil-sealed packets. Posterior packs may be constructed from a gauze roll (Figure 7.1) 4 cm long and 2 cm in diameter. A long, heavy silk suture is passed through one end of the roll, and the ends are left with equal length. Another silk ligature is tied firmly around the center of the roll, and the ends are again left long. Avoid excessively large packs that will block both choanae and force the patient to breathe through his mouth. Large packs also obstruct the eustachian tube and can lead to early otitis.

TECHNIQUE

Although the technique to be described is a proper one for determining the source of bleeding and treating it, it is in fact unnecessary for the majority of nosebleeds. Many anterior nosebleeds are allowed to continue for an inordinate length of time because the patient does not know how to treat himself. If the quantity and duration of flow do not suggest the need for formal cauterization, have the patient sit up and blow his nose to free it of clots. Grasp the nose between the thumb and forefinger and *squeeze it firmly for a full 5 minutes, by the clock.* This simple procedure applies pressure against Kiesselbach's plexus, the

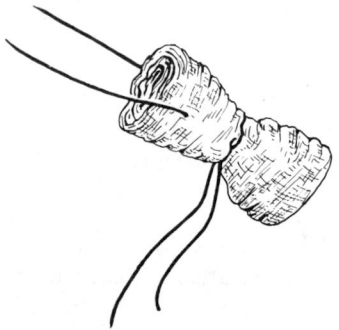

Figure 7.1.

Construction of a posterior nasal pack. One stitch is tied about the middle of the pack, and a second passes through the anterior portion.

anterior portion of the nasal septum from which the majority of hemorrhages originate, and it will stop most anterior nosebleeds.

If bleeding persists or recurs, a more thorough examination and treatment are indicated. Both patient and examiner should preferably be gowned and, unless there is evidence of shock, the patient should be comfortably seated. This posture avoids choking on pharyngeal blood in the recumbent position. A light is placed beside the patient's head and the head mirror is adjusted to throw a bright spot on the nose. Although blood may be present in both nasal passages, it is reasonable to assume that it originates from one side and one site only. Blood clots are blown free by the patient or aspirated, and the anterior septum is inspected with the nasal speculum for bleeding points. Occasionally, anterior hemorrhage springs from the anterior end of the inferior turbinate. If a bleeding source is located, a small cotton ball soaked in 1:1000 epinephrine solution is applied against it, and the nose squeezed to apply pressure for a full 5 minutes. The vessel is then cauterized with silver nitrate or the electric cautery. Use of the latter requires topical anesthesia with either 5% cocaine or 2% Pontocaine. The patient is warned to avoid picking or wiping the nose.

Anterior packing is reserved for bleeding that is difficult to stop or that is thought likely to recur. The petrolatum-impregnated packing is gently fed into the nostril with the bayonet forceps, placing the deep layers as far posterior as possible, then building the packing with sequentially more superficial ones.

If a bleeding site cannot be located, it may be presumed to be posterior in location. Because posterior bleeding usually comes from larger vessels (branches of the internal maxillary artery or the anterior ethmoidal artery), the hemorrhage is also generally more profuse, and the origin difficult to see, even with good light and suction.

The proper treatment of a posterior nosebleed is the placement of a posterior pack and an anterior pack in the affected side (Figure 7.2). A no. 14 gauge French rubber catheter is introduced through the bleeding nostril and led

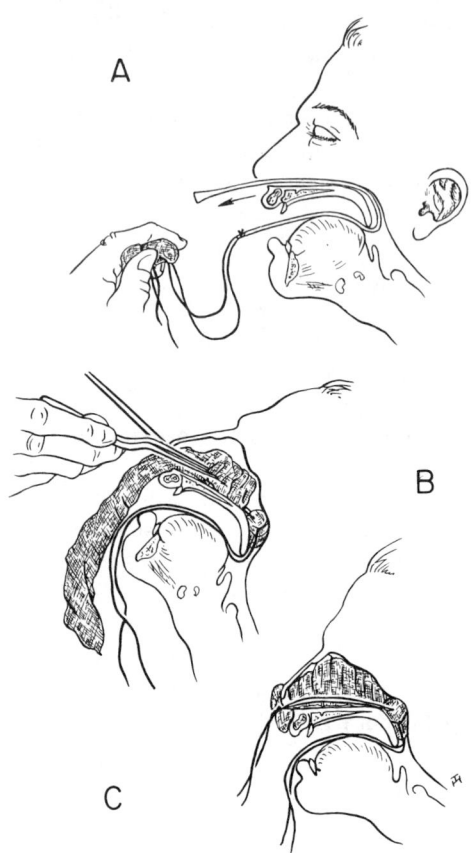

Figure 7.2.

Insertion of a posterior nasal pack. (**A**) The tie through the anterior portion of the pack is pulled into the choana by a red rubber catheter, and the tie about the center is allowed to hang out the mouth. (**B**) While tension is maintained on the stitch through the pack, anterior packing is introduced with bayonet forceps. (**C**) Anterior and posterior packing in place. The stitch through the posterior pack is tied about a separate gauze at the nose to maintain tension. The long ends of the tie about the middle of the pack are left to allow removal of the pack.

out the mouth. One end of the heavy suture through the posterior pack is fed through the opening in the catheter and is then tied to the other end to form a loop. The catheter is withdrawn out of the nose until resistance is felt as the pack enters the choana. The tie around the center of the pack is allowed to hang out of the mouth, and will later be tied in a loop. Traction on it is employed to dislodge and to remove the pack.

The ligature protruding from the nose is cut loose from the catheter, but gentle tension is maintained on it while an anterior pack is placed. The two ends of this ligature are then tied under light tension about a piece of gauze against the columella. A posterior pack is uncomfortable for the patient as long as it is in place, and it is usually removed after 3 or 4 days. A daily otoscopic examination should be performed to check for the development of otitis media or a hemorrhagic otitis. Obstruction of the sinus ostia can also lead to an acute sinusitis. Many otolaryngologists recommend prophylactic antibiotic therapy for all patients with posterior nasal packs, and for those with anterior packs in place for longer than 24 hours.

8.

NASOGASTRIC INTUBATION

One of the most common procedures performed in the hospital, nasogastric intubation is of great therapeutic and diagnostic value on the surgical, medical, and emergency room floors. The uses of this simple device are too numerous to list, but as any house officer or medical student with bile-stained sleeves can attest, its passage is not always accomplished with ease; there are an equal number of watery-eyed patients who can corroborate this. Although individual gag reflexes vary markedly, and there are a few who simply cannot tolerate anything touching their posterior pharynx, the method below will usually succeed in a reasonably smooth intubation.

MATERIAL
Levin tube (no. 16 French for adults and no. 12 French for children), water-soluble lubricant, tape of 1-inch width, regular type, Hoffman or other suitable small clamp, 50-ml syringe, catheter adapter if syringe does not have catheter tip, glass of water with a straw, emesis basin.

Comment. If there is a ward or wards on which gastric tubes are frequently used, a permanent list of the proper equipment should be left at the nurse's station. Of all the many experimental tubes for nasogastric intubation, the standard Levin tube remains the most useful. Made either of hard rubber or plastic, each type has its advocates. The latter is somewhat stiffer and hence easier to pass. Regardless of type chosen, however, request that it be iced for additional rigidity. The plastic Sheridan Salem or Andersen sump nasogastric tubes offer the theoretical advantage of an air break to prevent mucosal plugging of the drainage lumen. They require the availability of a constant suction apparatus, and they are not totally proof against blockage.

TECHNIQUE

Cooperation is of great importance. The patient will be fearful of an unpleasant experience if he has never been intubated before, and if he has, he will know he is in for an unpleasant experience. The common reactions to intubation, gagging, retching, and tearing of the eyes, are better tolerated if explained in advance, particularly when it is made clear that these discomforts are transient. Approach the patient with confidence and reasonable empathy, and reassure him of the necessity and value of this procedure. If the patient trusts the doctor, the battle is literally half won.

An assistant is essential, to perform two functions: holding the water, and if necessary (with children or confused patients), holding the patient. The patient should be in bed in a comfortable semisitting position, head slightly back and supported. Almost invariably, water is useful in passing a nasogastric tube. The reason is clear if anyone tries to swallow three times in rapid succession with no fluid in his mouth. It is extremely difficult. Even patients totally obstructed or about to undergo surgery may use water to help pass a Levin tube, simply because this fluid will be removed at once. The unconscious patient is, of course, an exception, but tests requiring a fasting stomach are not. The tube may be placed early, aspirated, and left in position off drainage.

Hands should be washed, but gloves are unnecessary. Lubricate the tip and the first few inches of the tube liberally, and tell the assistant to place the straw between the patient's lips. Instruct him not to drink, however, until so ordered, and then to drink as fast as possible *without stop-*

ping. This is an effective way to prevent coughing and gagging. While holding the tube, briefly inspect the nostrils for obvious deviations. Pass the tube gently along the floor of the nasal passageway. This is almost directly posterior (Figure 8.1). A common mistake is to push the tip both posterior and superior, losing it in the turbinates and causing pain and bleeding. Occasionally a hidden occlusion will necessitate changing to the opposite side.

When the tube begins to curve downward in the pharynx, and this is palpable, tell the patient firmly to drink and *keep drinking,* advancing the tip into the stomach as he swallows.

The average distance from the teeth to the esophagogastric junction in the adult is 45 cm, and most nasogastric tubes are marked at this point, and then at regular intervals thereafter. However, this distance varies considerably with build, and the single most reliable indication that the tube has advanced sufficiently is the rapid return of gastric contents on aspiration. It is best to advance well beyond the 45-cm

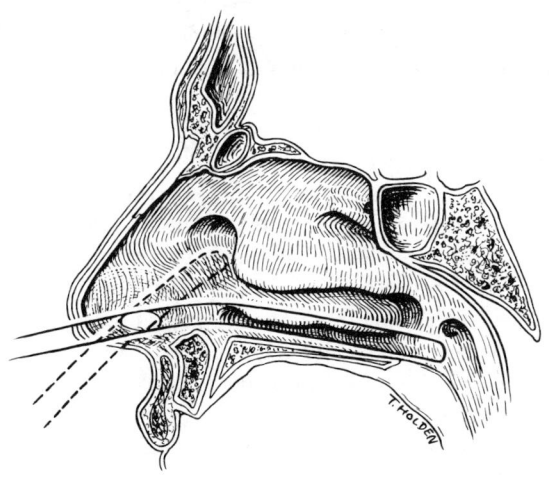

Figure 8.1.

Proper intranasal course for a nasogastric tube. The tube passes almost directly backward along the floor of the nasal passage, not superiorly, as indicated by the dotted lines.

mark, then slowly withdraw with aspiration until the best location is apparent. Another method to check position is rapidly to push in 20 ml of air with a syringe, while listening over the stomach with a stethoscope for the typical bubbling sound. If the patient gags and retches excessively, the tube may be curled up in his pharynx; this mishap can be checked simply by looking in his mouth. If the tip should pass inadvertently into the trachea, the breath will take on a characteristically hollow sound, and the patient will cough and will be unable to phonate properly. On occasion, the tip will become stuck in the esophagus, particularly in the presence of organic disease such as hiatus hernia, esophagitis, or malignant stricture. This initially may be confusing, because swallowed fluid will come back via the tube. However, the quantity returned will be slight, and if air is forced down into the tube, it will be heard bubbling in the pharynx, or the patient will belch almost immediately. This type of obstruction may often be passed by having the patient swallow more fluid while advancing once again. Once it is in position, secure the tube with a single, vertically split piece of 1-inch tape (Figure 8.2), in such a manner that it does not rest continuously against the edge of the nostrils. Prolonged contact here can cause eventual pressure necrosis, particularly in children.

From time to time it will be necessary to gavage or intubate an unconscious patient. If an overdose is suspected, it is much wiser to use the larger no. 32 French rubber tube, lubricated and passed through the mouth, for effective gavage and aspiration of stomach contents that might include solid food. When passing a nasogastric tube, a gloved hand palpating and guiding the tube as it passes down the posterior pharyngeal wall can be of great help. If the patient is comatose, his cough reflex may be depressed, and there will be little warning that the tube is passing into the trachea. Place the open end of the tube in a glass of water, and if it bubbles freely, the tip is probably within the trachea. Never irrigate the tube until certain that the tip is within the stomach walls. Airway intubation prior to gastric intubation will minimize the danger of tracheal aspiration.

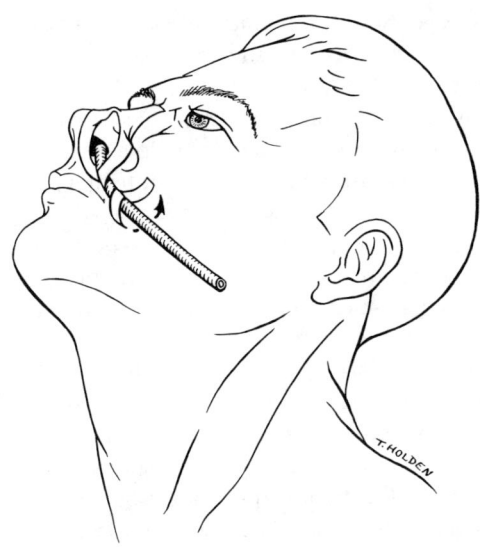

Figure 8.2.

The tube is held in position by a single piece of vertically split adhesive tape, placed to prevent either pressure or rubbing of the tube against the rim of the nostril.

It is a common belief that the presence of a nasogastric tube decreases a patient's pulmonary function, but this condition is of major significance only in those who already have severely compromised pulmonary reserve. If there is clear indication for gastric decompression, the status of the lungs should be disregarded except to be noted as an indication for vigorous pulmonary toilet. This is a necessity for any patient with chronic lung disease, with or without a nasogastric tube. The irritation and dryness secondary to the presence of this foreign body in the pharynx may rarely induce the "surgical parotitis" seen in the postoperative patient on prolonged nasogastric suction. It should be immediately suspected in any such patient who begins to complain of pain and tenderness about the angle of the jaw, and because the consequences of full-blown parotitis are severe morbidity and occasional mortality, the diagnosis is a clear indication for tube removal and therapy. This complication can usually be avoided, however, by meticulous mouth care and by allowing the patient to have an occasional sip of water around the tube.

A sip of water is in fact nothing more than an acceptable alternate way of irrigating the tube, and is feasible even when the most delicate anastomosis is under protection, *if the tube is draining properly* and quantity is restricted to sips. Nasogastric tubes and their suction devices require frequent observation and testing to maintain their smooth performance. Often manipulation of the tip of the catheter a few millimeters in either direction will convert absent drainage to adequate drainage. If there is difficulty in removing a nasogastric tube via the nose, the tube should be grasped via the mouth and checked for knotting. Children adapt themselves to nasogastric tubes rather slowly and tend to be stimulated to swallow by their presence. Complications such as laryngeal edema, sinusitis, and pharyngeal or esophageal erosion occur with greater frequency in this population, and the pediatric patient must be watched particularly for the development of otitis media.

The very unusual patient who seems unable to tolerate a Levin tube because of continuous retching and gagging may often be helped by additional sedation, but a stormy preoperative course should give the surgeon reason to consider a drainage gastrostomy if there is an abdominal operation scheduled.

Long Tubes

In recent years the frequency of use of long gastrointestinal tubes for bowel decompression in most medical centers has dropped steadily. The reasons are clear. Mechanical obstruction severe enough to cause the kind of distension for which long tubes are designed in the vast majority of cases also warrants surgical correction. The time required to feed such a device down the small intestines can delay the operation unnecessarily. There are now available several methods by which bowel may be rapidly decompressed intraoperatively, making this rather laborious preparation unnecessary and undesirable. The recurrence rate in patients obstructed by adhesive bands, in whom surgery is sometimes avoided by the use of such a tube, is so high as to discourage surgeons from its use as definitive management except in the extremely high-risk individual. In those patients with postoperative adynamic ileus who theoretically might benefit the most from the application of a long tube, the absence of propulsive peristalsis makes it extremely difficult to advance the tube properly, and air often reaccumulates in proximal loops as the tip decompresses the distal ones.

If a long tube is to be used, the Miller-Abbott type, with separate lumens for irrigation and for inflation of the soft rubber balloon just proximal to the tip, is usually easier to pass into the duodenum than the Cantor tube, which has a single lumen, although its larger diameter (18 French vs. 16 French) makes the Miller-Abbott tube more uncomfortable. This tube is passed in the same manner as the Levin tube, after first freely lubricating the collapsed balloon. The wall is marked at 45, 60, and 75 cm, and then at regular intervals up to 7 feet. When the tip is well within the stomach, the balloon is inflated with 15 to 20 ml of water. Mercury is *not* necessary and actually impedes its progress through the stomach. To facilitate passage into the duodenum and jejunum, the patient is now put through a series of maneuvers: he remains (1) semisitting for one hour on his left side; (2) right side down and slightly prone with feet elevated for two hours; (3) semisitting, then (4) lying on left side for one hour each. In reconstructing mentally the anatomy and posterior-anterior relationships of the stomach and duodenum, one will see that this rather mysterious rite becomes a logical effort to assist the passage of the Miller-Abbott tube through the stomach and duodenum by gravity. During this period, the tube is allowed to move freely, and at its conclusion, its position is checked fluoroscopically. Theoretically, it should have progressed into the jejunum. In practice, it will perhaps have entered the duodenum.

It is also possible to guide the tube directly into the duodenum by putting the patient through the maneuvers just mentioned in more rapid sequence, while gently advancing the tip. Once into the jejunum, the tube may be advanced about 10 cm per hour. To prevent inadvertent traction by the confused patient, tape the tube to the nose in the usual manner each time after advancing the tube; in alert patients the tube will advance more freely if left untaped. Because long tubes can easily tie themselves into knots that prevent either advancement or removal, it is unwise to push extra tubing into the gastric lumen. The lumen leading to the balloon should be firmly sealed and marked to prevent the mistake of accidental irrigation and inflation of the balloon while in the confines of the small bowel. Frequent irrigations and high intermittent suction aid the passage of this tube through distended bowel loops.

There are two accepted ways of removing a long tube. (1) The commonly applicable approach is to deflate the balloon completely, then to apply gentle traction on the tube until about 10 cm have been withdrawn at the nose, then to re-tape it and return hourly to repeat the process until it is totally removed. *Under no circumstances should any method of constant traction be employed.* It is quite easy to gather the jejunum like an accordion around the tip of the tube and perforate it in several places. (2) If there is difficulty in removing the tube in a retrograde manner, and if there is strong x-ray evidence that the tip has passed the area of obstruction, the tube may simply be cut at the nose and allowed to pass per rectum. The first method, however, should always be tried first. The occasional appearance of the tip of a Miller-Abbott tube protruding from the anus while the other end is still firmly attached at the nose is dramatic evidence of the extent to which the bowel may be gathered up upon the tube, even when passing smoothly.

Sengstaken-Blakemore Tube
This tube was designed and is effective for the treatment of a single condition: control of bleeding esophageal varices. Although cessation of bleeding with this tube is presumptive evidence that upper gastrointestinal bleeding is in fact coming from varices, particularly if it recurs when the balloons are released, duodenal ulcers may stop bleeding while a patient has one of these tubes in place, and every

effort should be made by esophagoscopy, gastroscopy, and barium studies to arrive at a firm diagnosis *before the tube is passed.*

There are detailed instructions for use that accompany each tube, and these instructions should be consulted. Essentially, the Sengstaken-Blakemore tube is a triple-lumen rubber tube with two balloons, a round gastric balloon and a tubular esophageal balloon, and one lumen for gastric aspiration, all openings into the tube being distal to the gastric balloon. The tube is necessarily large, and nasal passage is uncomfortable. In addition, if the patient is awake and alert, sedation should be employed while the tube is inflated, both for comfort and for reduction of the incidence of retching and regurgitation. Always use a new tube. After checking the balloons for leaks, the tube is generously lubricated and passed through the nose in the usual manner until the 50-cm mark on the wall is reached. Gastric contents are aspirated. The gastric balloon is next inflated with 100 to 200 ml of air, and the tube pulled back until resistance is felt. With slight tension, the tube is held in place against the nostril by means of a sponge rubber cuff taped around it at this point. Care should be taken to avoid potentially necrosing pressure here. An alternate method of securing the tube with proper tension is to tape it to the face mask of a standard football helmet. The esophageal balloon is next inflated to 35 to 40 mHg pressure by a standard aneroid gauge manometer, and the stomach copiously lavaged with cold saline solution for one-half hour or until clear. If it does not clear, pressure in the esophageal tamponade may be increased to 45 mHg, and the lavage repeated. Higher pressures are not recommended, and even this degree may cause considerable discomfort. Also, failure to gain control at this pressure should lead one to reconsider the diagnosis.

If splenic pulp pressures have previously been determined, they can serve as a guide for intraesophageal settings, but they are not always reliable. Esophageal contractions, respiratory movements, coughing, and retching can cause wide fluctuations in the intraesophageal balloon pressure, with peaks as high as 70 mHg not being unusual. The pressure should be checked regularly at 30-minute to 60-minute intervals for leaks, but baseline intraluminal pressure is the only important pressure to maintain constant, and transient peaks will not affect the efficiency of the tube. After total evacuation, the stomach is placed on constant drainage for 12 to 24 hours, after which time gastric feedings by way of the tube may be started. Should the bleeding continue at the higher intraesophageal tamponade pressure, the gastric balloon may be inflated to 300 or 400 ml of air for temporary control of presumed gastric varices. Inasmuch as this pressure may well ulcerate the gastric mucosa within 6 hours, the step should be considered only as preparation for surgery.

After hemorrhage is controlled, the pressure within the esophageal balloon is lowered until the lowest point is reached that still prevents bleeding, and this is then maintained for 48 hours. The esophageal and gastric balloons are then deflated over a period of 6 to 8 hours, and left in position for another 24 hours. If bleeding recurs, the balloons should be immediately reinflated and maintained for an additional 48 hours. Bleeding after two attempts at control with a Sengstaken-Blakemore tube is rarely controlled with a third try; if this condition occurs, the patient should be considered for emergency surgery, either a portosystemic shunt or a direct attack on the varices. Criteria for acceptability are not standardized, and are beyond the purposes of this book, but they include the general state of the patient and the functional capacity of the liver. Hepatic coma and inability to raise the prothrombin time to acceptable levels are generally acknowledged contraindications to surgery.

The use of this tube carries certain inherent hazards for the patient, and repeatedly, clinical series describing its effectiveness also list major tube-related morbidity and mortality in excess of 15 percent. The complications most often reported are (1) rupture or erosion of the esophagus, (2) dislocation of the esophageal balloon with airway obstruction, and (3) aspiration. There are several safeguards against these potentially fatal side effects which should become standard operating principles whenever a Blakemore-Sengstaken tube is passed. The nasopharynx should not be anesthetized. A small nasogastric tube should be passed through the other nostril and positioned above the esophageal balloon to aspirate swallowed saliva. For the unconscious patient, a complementary tracheostomy may be necessary to prevent aspiration. Inflation of the gastric balloon with at least 200 ml of air will prevent it from riding up into the esophagus and thereby allowing the esophageal balloon to produce airway obstruction. Limit the patient's exposure to fully inflated balloon pressure to 48 hours.

Feeding Catheters

Plastic, prepackaged feeding tubes, usually no. 8 French size, are readily available and are useful adjuncts in the treatment of many chronic illnesses requiring supplemental oral intake or total control of feeding. The viscosity of most feeding mixtures renders tubes of smaller caliber impractical. However, the inherent flexibility of a catheter this small, and its tendency to curl in the pharynx, often makes it difficult to pass these tubes into the stomach. The following simple step can avoid the problem in most cases.

The tip of the feeding tube and the tip of a standard nasogastric tube are squeezed together into the empty half of a large gelatin capsule, such as any of the larger barbiturate capsules. The tubes and capsule are lubricated, and the entire combination is passed as a unit through the nose into the stomach, as described at the beginning of this chapter. Within one-half hour, the capsule will have dissolved, and the larger tube may be removed, leaving the feeding tube taped in place and undisturbed.

A well-lubricated ureteral catheter, passed full length into the feeding tube, will also give it the required stiffness to pass easily. Test the catheter for ease of withdrawal before attempting this maneuver.

9.

LUMBAR PUNCTURE

Too frequently lumbar puncture is a procedure learned by interns from interns. Incorrect techniques and inadequate safety precautions are passed from generation to generation, until a disaster points out that "getting by" is not good enough. Observing a lumbar puncture performed by an experienced neurologist or neurosurgeon is an invaluable experience, and the first attempt should be with such expert assistance. In this manner, patient comfort and safety will benefit, and the yield of information will improve.

A local infection near the site of the proposed puncture is a recognized contraindication to lumbar puncture, but it should also be remembered that meningitis can follow a spinal tap performed on patients with septicemia, presumably from organisms picked up by the needle passing through the tissues of the back. Whenever feasible, such infection should be well under control before a lumbar puncture is attempted.

The suspected presence of any space-occupying lesion in the head causing increased cerebrospinal pressure (and cerebrovascular lesions can function in this manner during the phase of acute swelling) must lead one to weigh the risk of brain herniation versus the value of the information gained. Marked papilledema and posterior fossa neoplasms are generally accepted as contraindications to lumbar tap, but the neurosurgical staff should be consulted in borderline instances. Whenever possible, lumbar puncture should precede myelography or pneumoencephalography by one week.

MATERIAL

Sterilized lumbar puncture set: manometer, 5-ml syringe, 25-gauge and 22-gauge needles, 20-gauge and 22-gauge spinal needles, three-way stopcock, 3 culture and fluid collection tubes, sponges, dressing towels, ampules of local anesthetic. Floor supplies: sterile gloves, mask, antiseptic-soaked sponges.

Comment. Prepackaged, sterilized, disposable lumbar puncture trays are widely available and generally satisfactory.

TECHNIQUE

Discuss the nature of the procedure with the patient and reassure him about its safety and lack of discomfort, because he frequently will have heard tales about spinal headaches and neurological disasters. An assistant is of great help.

The patient lies on his side, with his back at the edge of the bed (Figure 9.1), and the operator is seated comfortably facing the back. To open up the intervertebral spaces posteriorly, request that he flex his back as much as possible. The assistant can aid him in this by standing on the opposite side of the bed, or kneeling on it, and, while supporting the patient behind his knees, pressing firmly downward with his free arm placed over the patient's neck. This maneuver is particularly effective in children.

Although the sitting position allows the lumbar interspinous spaces to spread more than in the lateral position, punctures so performed are more dangerous, more likely to be followed by headache, and are unsatisfactory for dynamics. It should be used only when the lateral position has proved unsatisfactory, and in experienced hands *this situation is very unusual.*

Using a strict aseptic technique, place a sterile towel on the bed underneath the patient (the operator folds the towel

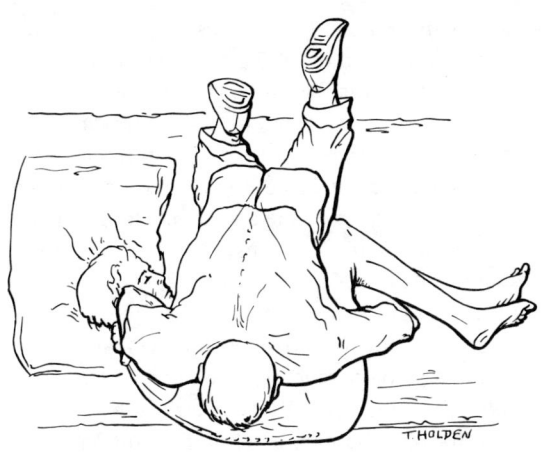

Figure 9.1.

Proper fetal position for lumbar puncture. An assistant kneels on the bed and places his right arm behind the patient's neck, and his left arm beneath the patient's buttocks. Pressure can be exerted by him to increase or maintain the amount of flexion of the lumbar spine.

over his gloves, pushes the edge of the fold beneath the back, then removes his hands), and fold another along the upper edge of the back. Cleanse the back carefully, working outward in a spiral fashion from the site of the proposed puncture, but widely enough to include several interspaces.

The most common sites selected for lumbar puncture are the L3–L4 interspace, or the L4–L5 interspace, to ensure being below the level of the spinal cord (in adults the lowest level is usually L1, but in infants and young children the cord may be injured as low as the L2–L3 interspace). The L3–L4 interspace lies at the level of the posterior iliac crests, and a suitable puncture site may be chosen by palpating the iliac crest through the upper towel, selecting a midline spot at this level, and then choosing the nearest interspace. Determine the midline by palpation of the spine, not by the location of the gluteal crease. In an obese patient the skin may sag considerably when he turns, and this crease can then be well off center.

A wheal of local anesthesia is raised at this site, and infiltration carried down between the spinous processes of the L3–L4 vertebrae. The spinal needle, with stylet in place, is now introduced through the wheal, but not at the precise point where the skin was punctured by the infiltrating needle; this precaution is to prevent picking up red cells from the earlier puncture. To avoid introduction of foreign material, never touch the tip of the spinal needle, and whisk free any gauze threads that might cling to it from the kit. Hold the spinal needle like a pencil, with the index finger securing the stylet in place; insert it as near as possible to the superior border of the lower spinous process; and advance slowly in a plane parallel with the bed and with a 30-degree cephalad inclination. Advance until the "give" of the ligamentum flavum, then the arachnoid membrane, are felt, and withdraw the stylet. These structures are not always clearly palpable, and unless the operator is experienced, he would be wise to remove the stylet intermittently while advancing it. Turn the needle so that the wound of entrance in the dura will be vertical rather than horizontal (the latter will tend to leak more). If the needle tip is felt to be in the subarachnoid space, but no fluid is forthcoming, slowly rotate the needle in both directions—if the tip is truly through the dura, this maneuver should not enlarge the tear. The stylet may be replaced, and the needle advanced a short distance, if this rotation is unsuccessful. Should fluid still not appear, the tip should be withdrawn *to the subcutaneous tissue* before checking landmarks and attempting a new pass. Insufficient withdrawal will result in the needle following the original path.

When bone is encountered (Figure 9.2), estimation of its depth from the skin will assist in selecting a proper new angle of passage. If bone is encountered at a shallow depth, increase the angle; if at a medium depth, decrease the angle; if overly deep, the needle is off the midline. It may prove helpful to avoid previous blind paths by leaving the needle in place as a guide, then selecting another for the new attempt. Three passes constitute a reasonable effort, and severe osteoarthritis may require an effort at another interspace.

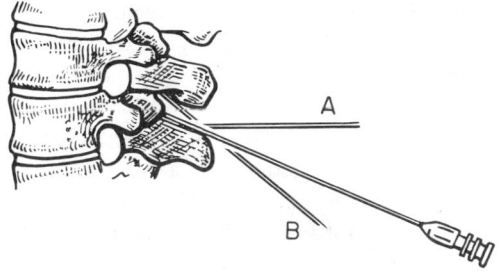

Figure 9.2.

(**A**) When bone is encountered at a shallow depth, redirecting the needle in a more cephalad direction is indicated. (**B**) When bone is encountered at a deeper level, redirecting the needle in a more caudal direction may help.

When increased intracranial pressure is suspected, initial removal of the stylet should be performed cautiously, to avoid a sudden gush of cerebrospinal fluid. A falsely elevated initial pressure may be caused by patient tension, or by the simple fact that the patient's head may be elevated above the level of the puncture by a pillow or an uneven mattress. Congestive heart failure, ascites, asthma, and vena cava syndromes also elevate pressure artifactually. When the needle is in place, tell the patient that he can relax and can expect no more discomfort. Opening pressure should be measured with a manometer. Pressure over 180 mm is abnormal. Dynamics then follow, but these are indicated only if there is a question of a block in the spinal canal, with definite signs or symptoms referable to structures above the foramen magnum. A large needle (preferably an 18-gauge, but a 20-gauge is acceptable), is desirable for dynamics. Once this needle is properly positioned, pressure on the abdomen, or a Queckenstedt test (manual compression of both internal jugular veins), will cause a rapid rise in cerebrospinal fluid pressure by increasing pressure in the veins flowing out of the spinal space. This will not occur in the presence of a block in the subarachnoid space above the level of the puncture. A rise of less than 100 mm of water, however, is difficult to interpret.

Note. Because a partial block in the cervical region may not be apparent in certain positions of the head, dynamics should be evaluated with the head flexed, neutral, and extended.

Cerebrospinal fluid is removed for indicated chemical, bacteriologic, and morphologic studies, and a closing pressure is recorded after noting the amount of fluid withdrawn. To avoid trapping a nerve root against the spinal needle, cerebrospinal fluid is never aspirated, but is allowed to run freely. The needle is withdrawn, and a small sterile bandage is applied over the puncture site.

When the initial return is bloody, the color of the supernate should be noted after centrifugation of the sample. Xanthochromia suggests pretap hemorrhage. A careful cell count, before and after lysis of the red blood cells with glacial acetic acid, should be done, together with a count of total cells in the first and last tubes. Comparison of the ratio of red cells to white cells in the spinal fluid with that in the peripheral blood will help to differentiate true subarachnoid hemorrhage from a traumatic puncture. Remember that patients with true subarachnoid bleeding can have traumatic taps. This invalidates the old saw that blood from a traumatic puncture clears as the collection continues.

The problem of spinal headaches is a difficult one. The occurrence of these headaches has been correlated only with the size of the needle and the excitement attending the actual puncture. Because the incidence of headache decreases with the use of smaller needles, the use of a 22-gauge spinal needle is adequate and preferable in routine punctures without dynamics. It is also wise to keep the patient prone for the first hour, in bed for 6 to 12 hours, and to force fluids for the first 24 hours. In order to spare him a full day in bed, plan the puncture for the early evening if feasible. Headache may be delayed in appearance for up to one week. They are better accepted if the patient has been prepared for their possibility in advance.

Within 12 hours of a previous lumbar puncture, the cerebrospinal fluid pressure will ordinarily not be affected enough by leakage to render a subsequent effort too difficult. A 24-hour delay, however, may make it necessary to use the negative pressure of the epidural space (causing a bubble in the hub of the needle to be sucked inward), as an indication of proper location.

The fluid cell count should be done by the operator. Remember that, without stains, the differentiation of cell types is difficult even in expert hands.

Before the puncture, check the volume requirements of the laboratories for the studies desired. Refrigerate an extra milliliter of sterile cerebrospinal fluid as a reserve. Sugar, chloride, and protein levels (this last may be roughly indicated by the use of a standard dipstick reagent), as well as bacterial cultures should be performed on all spinal fluid samples.

10.

URETHRAL CATHETERIZATION

Patients with both abnormal and normal genitourinary tracts may require urethral catheterization. In the latter category are those patients with postoperative retention, gynecologic and obstetric patients, patients in shock or being monitored for major cardiovascular surgery, victims of strokes or accidents, and many others for whom eventual return to completely normal function is anatomically feasible. Safe and gentle dexterity with the urethral catheter is essential if this feasibility is to become a probability.

Although properly implicated as the source of serious urinary tract infection, the catheter is also unquestionably an instrument of great therapeutic value, and hesitancy in its use when indicated can lead to infections and morbidity of even more serious consequences. In borderline situations, a fine sense of clinical balance is often required, a judgment born of repeated experience. Perhaps the most frustrating problem of all is postoperative retention.

Postoperative catheterization should be avoided until conservative measures have been afforded a reasonable trial. One of the most useful conservative measures is simply to make certain that the patient has voided before leaving for the operating room. What constitutes a reasonable postoperative trial period will be somewhat dependent upon the vigor of the postoperative hydration, but in general, if the patient has not voided within 12 to 14 hours after the induction of anesthesia, it is unlikely that he will do so adequately thereafter, and the odds diminish with time.

It is unnatural for a man to void in the supine position, and unless contraindicated, his first efforts should be made at least in the sitting position, and standing with support if possible. When it is known that the patient will not be able to stand postoperatively, he should practice voiding into a urinal in bed before surgery. Women may often be allowed bathroom privileges the evening after many operations if the facilities and nurses are nearby. Common sense will dictate this decision, *with the degree of postoperative sedation as the key variable.* In general, patients should not attempt to void during the peak effect of analgesics and sedatives, and those requiring large amounts will uniformly have the greatest difficulties. Psychological factors are important in any voluntary act, and the unduly anxious patient should be specifically reassured and relaxed about his first attempts. The sound of running water and the scent of oil of wintergreen are but two of a host of ancient methods to assist the patient's own volition. In this regard, do not neglect simple privacy. A man propped up against the side of his bed, with one hand holding the urinal and the other over the shoulder of an attractive nurse, is facing obstacles that would stagger Freud himself. Even in the recovery room he may be allowed the seclusion of drawn bed curtains, and if it seems unwise to leave him unguarded, a male nurse or attendant should be present.

Skill in managing these conservative aids will reduce the need for postoperative catheterizations. Should they fail, the parasympathomimetic drug Urecholine, given as a single 5-mg subcutaneous injection, will often result in adequate evacuation within 15 minutes, thus affording a period of grace until the following morning, when chances of spontaneous success are greater. Side effects that include cramps, vomiting, dizziness, and sweating are common with the parenteral use of this drug, and in any condition in which parasympathetic stimulation might be dangerous (asthma, coronary artery disease, heart block, fresh gastrointestinal or vesical suture lines), the drug is dangerous. Its use is absolutely contraindicated in the presence of suspected gastrointestinal or urethral obstruction.

If these measures have proved fruitless, be bold in the decision to catheterize. Allowing the bladder to become grossly overdistended will obviate any chance for normal micturition and will entail the risk of prolonged dysfunction and infection. It has been the feeling of many physicians that once a catheter is required, it is better to leave it in place until the patient is up and about. Although a single catheterization and removal admittedly will sometimes suffice, the risk of infection from repeated catheterizations outweighs the hazard of having the patient remain for 24 to 48 hours on a properly attended indwelling tube. The question is not a settled one, and a compromise might be reached by using a Foley catheter and then basing the decision upon the amount of urine released (and hence the degree of distension), leaving in the catheter for volumes exceeding 350 or 400 ml.

MATERIAL
Sterile gloves, cleansing sponges (aqueous Zephiran solution or diluted pHisoHex are both excellent), sterile Foley catheter with 5-ml balloon (no. 14 French for women, no. 16 French for men), sterile towels and Kelly clamp, syringe with needle containing 5 ml saline solution, water-soluble lubricant (antibiotic-impregnated ones such as Neosporin offer some protection against inoculation with urethral organisms during catheterization), appropriate connecting tubing and collection bag (with an air break enclosed in the system), culture tube, sterile basin.

Comment. Prepackaged, sterile catheterization sets are now widely available and generally satisfactory. The catheter sizes mentioned above are the standard ones available in such sets. Do not catheterize a patient with an unduly large tube; this will cause early urethral irritation and inflammation.

TECHNIQUE

Male Catheterization

Allow the patient the maximum degree of privacy during this procedure. He should be in bed, supine or semisitting, with the contents of the opened catheterization tray within easy reach. Put on the gloves, after washing, and prepare the tray, including spreading the lubricant and placing a towel beneath the penis. If the foreskin is present, it should be stripped back gently with the left hand, which then holds the penile shaft, and any accumulated smegma should be washed off; it is necessary to cleanse only the glans. Use the sterile Kelly clamp or a forceps to hold the cleansing sponges, maintaining sterility of the right (or dominant) hand. To prevent retraction of the short penis, or contamination by the restless patient, do not let go of the penile shaft with the left hand.

Touch nothing but the catheter with the right hand, holding it in such a manner (Figure 10.1) that the flared

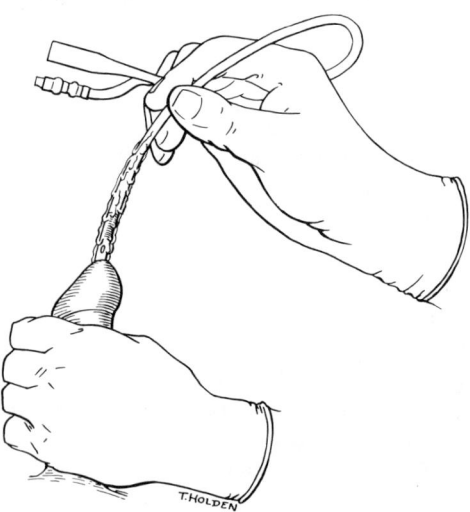

Figure 10.1.

Urethral catheterization. Left hand immobilizes and lifts penile shaft. As catheter progresses, it is allowed to slide through the fingers of the right hand; this hand touches nothing but the catheter.

end will not become contaminated. (In some prepackaged sets, the catheter is already connected to the drainage tubing—do not break this connection.) As long as the right hand remains sterile, the catheter may be advanced by the fingers. Lubricate the first several inches of the tip generously and place a small amount of lubrication about the meatus. Raise the shaft of the penis straight up with the left hand, thereby straightening the prostatic urethra. Introduce and pass the catheter rapidly, following the anterior wall of the urethra. There are two times the patient will commonly feel most discomfort during catheterization: as the tip enters the glans, and as it passes through the prostatic portion of the urethra. Even without significant prostatic obstruction, some resistance will be noticed as this latter area is reached. Maintain elevation and slight tension at this point to ease passage.

Advance the catheter almost to its bifurcation before inflating the balloon, to ensure against trapping the balloon in the urethra. The open end may be clamped to prevent leakage while the balloon is inflated. Withdraw the catheter slightly, and after securing a specimen for culture, connect it to the drainage system, at all times avoiding touching or contaminating the open end. If the patient complains of pain during inflation, or the catheter cannot be moved after inflation, it is incorrectly positioned and should be deflated. Tape the tubing, not the catheter, to the inner surface of the thigh in such a way that it prevents tension on the balloon (and thus the bladder neck) as the patient moves. Also, taping the tubing rather than the catheter will prevent the catheter from riding in and out of the urethra as he walks. *Note. Remember to reduce the foreskin.* Paraphimosis secondary to catheterizations in 99 percent of cases is a monument to simple negligence. The patient cannot be depended upon to remind the physician of this problem or to notice it until swelling may have reached proportions requiring a dorsal slit.

If the catheter cannot be passed after a short time, withdraw it. Undue persistence will result only in pain and muscle spasm that will make later attempts more difficult.

If there is no suspected obstruction, try a no. 14 or a no. 12 French Foley catheter (Figure 10.2A). Smaller sizes than these are usually too flexible. If this also fails, or if the patient has organic obstruction, secondary either to a urethral stricture or an enlarged prostate, the following maneuvers should be followed in a logical progression.

The urethra may be concomitantly lubricated and partially anesthetized by forcing into it a sterile aqueous jelly containing a topical anesthetic, such as Xylocaine. This anesthetic is supplied in a tube equipped with an acorn tip adapter that allows direct transfer into the urethra. An Asepto or standard medicinal syringe may also be used. Push in 10 to 15 ml of the jelly in a retrograde manner

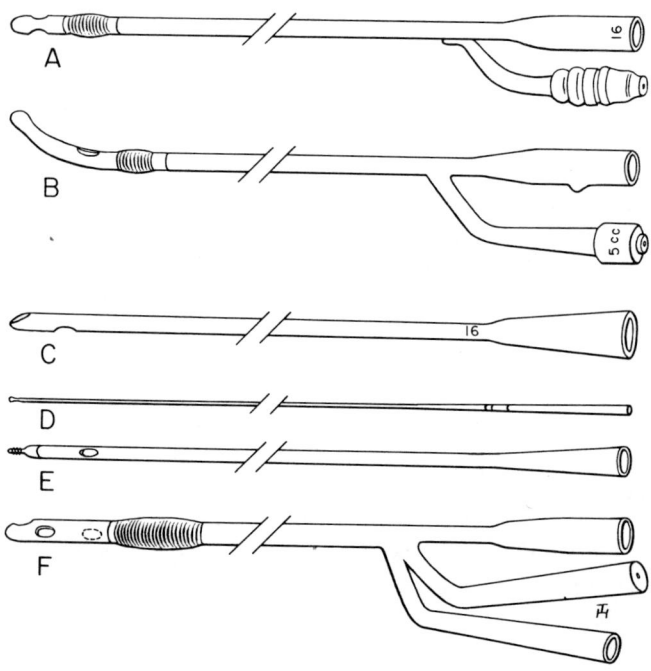

Figure 10.2.

Various urethral catheters. (**A**) Foley catheter. (**B**) Coudé-tip Foley catheter. (**C**) Straight catheter with "whistle tip." (**D**) Filiform. (**E**) Follower. (**F**) Three-way catheter for continuous irrigation of the bladder.

while constricting the glans about the nozzle with the free
hand. Raise the scrotum and massage the jelly into the
prostatic urethra for 30 seconds. Although lubrication is
the prime objective, the anesthetic is important not only to
relieve pain, but also to relax reflex muscle spasm. The
patient with acute retention may require sedation and
analgesia with morphine to achieve adequate relaxation.

Either a no. 14 or a no. 16 French straight catheter (Figure 10.2C) or Foley catheter may now be used to pass the
obstruction. The former possesses more inherent rigidity,
particularly if those made of Silastic are available. These
valuable instruments also have the added advantage of being
inert, and are therefore less prone to incite urethritis when
indwelling over 48 hours. If the patient is disoriented or
elderly, a straight catheter might well be the tube of choice
from the outset. A 5-ml balloon on a Foley catheter will
not offer full security against removal by the sharp tug of a
confused patient, thus exposing him to the risk of urethral
damage and a severe bout of septicemia. A straight catheter
must be taped in place, as illustrated in Figure 10.3, and
thus is not usually suitable for chronic drainage.

If a Foley catheter is tried again, pass a no. 7 or a no. 8
French ureteral catheter down its bore first. This will give it
considerably greater rigidity without the sacrifice of flexi-

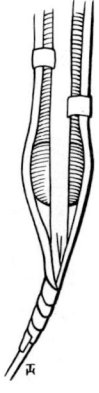

Figure 10.3.
Method of taping straight urethral catheter in place.

bility, or need for a larger gauge attendant upon the use of a stiff metal introducer.

Should these twin measures of increased urethral lubrication and stiffness of catheter both prove inadequate, and the obstruction seems to be in the prostatic urethra, a no. 14 or a no. 16 French coudé-tip rubber catheter may be tried (Figure 10.2B). This has a stiffly woven, angled tip designed specifically to pass the urethral bend at the prostate. The use of a larger no. 18 or no. 20 French Foley catheter, containing a stiff, lubricated metal stylet, curved in the shape of a urethral sound, is the final method for passing a severe prostatic obstruction, but the danger of forcing a false passage with such an instrument warrants its use only by those with considerable urologic experience. The stylet is lubricated to ensure its removability once the catheter is in place, and it should be tested for this before passage is attempted. Following the anterior wall of the urethra will lessen the danger of perforating its membranous portion.

Penile urethral strictures are best handled with filiforms and followers (Figures 10.2D, E). The slender, olive-tipped filiform is eased through the stricture into the bladder, and then the narrowed area is dilated as progressively larger followers are screwed into the filiform and passed along the same tract. Several filiforms should be on hand, for it is often necessary to introduce three or four sequentially and manipulate each until one finds the proper lumen. The largest catheter follower possible is then taped in place in the same manner as a straight catheter.

If the constriction of phimosis is severe enough to interfere with catheterization, temporary correction may be accomplished by a simple dorsal slit. The dorsal foreskin is anesthetized, a grooved director passed beneath it in the midline, and the foreskin divided longitudinally with a scalpel over the director. The inner and outer skin edges are sutured together. Phimosis of this degree warrants later circumcision.

Paraphimosis may also require a dorsal slit, but this condition usually can be sufficiently reduced by gentle, per-

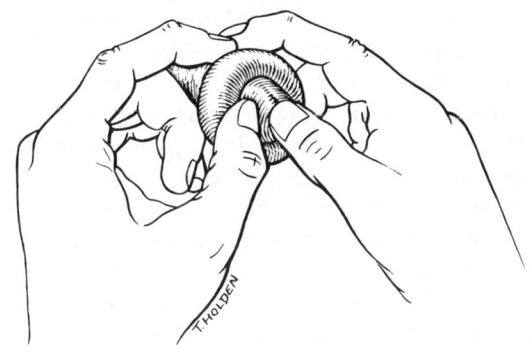

Figure 10.4.
Reduction of paraphimosis. Thumbs and forefingers are pressed together to "milk" subcutaneous fluid away from the glans.

sistent digital "milking" of the fluid away from the glans, followed by reduction of the foreskin (Figure 10.4).

Rapid decompression of a greatly distended bladder following catherization has been reported as a cause of shock, particularly in the elderly man. If the patient's clinical examination suggests severe distension, allow the urine to drain off in 400-ml increments, clamping the catheter intermittently for 15-minute periods until the bladder is emptied.

Female Catheterization

A female nurse should be present. Preparation is with the same solutions, the patient being supported by the nurse throughout the procedure in the supine position, with knees bent and hips abducted. The recessed position of the urethra makes it somewhat difficult to cleanse thoroughly. The high incidence of urinary tract infections in catheterized women is a direct result of breaks in technique at the time of catheter injection. Too frequently the task is assigned to a junior nurse with little experience, lighting is poor, and the catheter is dipped into several orifices before finding its way into the urethra. Review female genital anatomy, use a strong light, and make certain that the nurse retracts the labia adequately (and *keeps* them retracted) so that the urethral meatus can be adequately visualized and cleansed.

Urethral dilatation with metal sounds is done prior to catheterization if a stricture is present; otherwise, a no. 14 or no. 16 French Foley catheter is passed in the standard manner, again being taped to the leg so as to allow slack between the tape and urethral meatus. If the patient will require drainage for several days, as following a gynecologic procedure, a three-way catheter (see Figure 10.2F) that allows the constant infusion of an antibiotic-containing solution such as Neosporin may be selected in an effort to reduce the incidence of catheter-induced urinary-tract infections. Because of the constant infusion, these catheters are not recommended when careful monitoring of urinary output is critical.

Catheterization of Children

There are two special considerations when an indwelling catheter becomes necessary in children: (1) Do not try to force a catheter that is too large. (2) Make the use of a lubricant with a surface-active anesthetic, such as Xylocaine or Surfacaine, standard procedure.

Catheter Care

To prevent urinary tract infections in patients with indwelling catheters, vigil must be maintained against the introduction of organisms either along the catheter at the urethral meatus, or through the catheter, by inappropriate handling of the tubing.

A Zephiran- or Betadine-soaked dressing may be applied around the catheter at the meatus and changed twice daily in male patients. With women, and often with men too, an effective alternative is cleansing the meatal area with a Zephiran, pHisoHex, or Betadine sponge and carefully removing any encrustations. The patients may perform this task themselves, and if properly instructed and impressed with the importance of this ritual, they will prove highly motivated. Cleansing should be done three or four times a day; if the patient is confused or heavily sedated, this operation becomes the responsibility of the attending physician and nursing staff. On female wards, catheter care ideally should become a standard routine.

Drainage sets that incorporate the air break chamber in their tubing are widely available; these sets are uniformly preferable to those without this safety feature. In addition, nurses must be instructed in the proper handling of these sets. Samples for volume measurement, urinalysis, or electrolyte determinations are to be removed from the bag and *always distal to the drip chamber.* Urine distal to this chamber should be considered infected, and usually is. The collection bag, therefore, must never be allowed in a position that would allow retrograde flow of urine back into the bladder. If the catheter must be disconnected from the tubing to obtain a culture specimen, the strictest sterile technique is mandatory, neither open end is touched, and both ends are lavaged with an antiseptic before they are reconnected. Repeatedly such common-sense principles, when widely practiced, have sharply reduced the hospital incidence of catheter-induced infections.

Intermittent instillations of antiseptic solutions are advocated as another protection against infection, but they require the repeated opening, and hence possible contamination, of a closed drainage system. A terminal instillation of 50 ml of such a solution, just prior to removal of the catheter, is also frequently recommended.

SUPRAPUBIC INTRACATH OR NEEDLE DRAINAGE

When the bladder is overdistended, it is possible to achieve its satisfactory, if somewhat slow, decompression by passing a 14-gauge 2-inch Intracath into the bladder directly superior to the symphysis pubis. The skin is carefully prepared and shaved if necessary, and the site of the puncture anesthetized. Once the bladder is penetrated, the needle is withdrawn and the catheter connected to I.V. tubing and an empty solution bottle. This procedure might be chosen in an individual, such as a young man following elective surgery, when the desire not to catheterize is strong, or in the rare instance of urethral obstruction unamenable to relief from the usual techniques and in the absence of ready urologic assistance. The bladder *must* be clearly palpable above the pubis, and the Intracath *must* be removed immediately after decompression. Commercial puncture sets are also available.

A 20-gauge needle on a standard syringe may be used in a similar manner to obtain culture specimens in uncatheterized patients, particularly children, in whom the bladder occupies a higher position in relation to the public symphysis. The bladder must be made palpable, if necessary, by having the patient first drink a large quantity of water.

11.

DIALYSIS TECHNIQUES

11.1. PERITONEAL DIALYSIS

Although hemodialysis has largely replaced peritoneal dialysis for chronic management of patients with end-stage renal failure, peritoneal dialysis maintains a definite usefulness for patients whose renal failure is reversible or for interim management when hemodialysis might be difficult or contraindicated.

MATERIAL
Peritoneal dialysis catheter, prepackaged and sterile, such as the Trocath or Stylocath, and a 5-ml syringe with 25-gauge and 22-gauge needles, local anesthetic, no. 11 scalpel blade, scalpel handle, 4-0 silk, and sterile towels. Floor supplies: skin disinfectant, sterile gloves, dialysis fluid and administration set.

TECHNIQUE
The site usually chosen for peritoneal dialysis is the midline of the abdomen, approximately one-third of the distance from the umbilicus to the symphysis pubis. The patient is in the supine position, and the bladder should be emptied prior to beginning the procedure. Areas of previous abdominal incisions should be avoided, for bowel may be adherent to the peritoneum beneath them. Previous peritonitis also

increases the likelihood of adhesions. A distended abdomen makes peritoneal dialysis more hazardous. If the bowel is distended, the possibility of bowel perforation is enhanced, and if the abdomen is distended with ascitic fluid, a troublesome, persistent leak around the catheter will often occur.

The area where the catheter is to be inserted is prepared with disinfectant, and a skin wheal of local anesthetic is placed and infiltrated into the abdominal wall and down to the level of the peritoneum as well. A half-centimeter incision is made in the skin, and the catheter, with the stylet inserted, is introduced into the peritoneal cavity by a twisting motion, while the incision is held open with the thumb and index finger of the free hand. The patient is requested to tense his abdominal wall to assist in the perforation of the peritoneum. Once the peritoneum is punctured, the depth of penetration is controlled by grasping the catheter with the thumb and index finger. The tip of the stylet is withdrawn slightly and the catheter is angled caudally, then guided gently toward the right or left pelvic gutter and into a dependent portion of the abdominal cavity. A springy resistance to advancement usually indicates that the course of the catheter is extraperitoneal. The line should be withdrawn and a new stylet puncture made.

When all the catheter perforations are within the abdominal cavity, the L-shaped adapter is attached and dialysis fluid is allowed to enter the abdominal cavity. This instillation of fluid will assist in final placement of the catheter in the proper position. A single stitch is used to snug up the hole about the catheter, or this hole may be left open. A sterile dressing is applied to cover the area and to help maintain the proper position of the catheter. If the peritoneal catheter is too long, it may be cut and the L-shaped adapter repositioned.

To assist in full and even distribution of the dialysis fluid within the peritoneal cavity, the patient is turned from side to side during both the instillation and equilibrium phases of the peritoneal dialysis. Warming the solutions to 37° C or increasing the liters per hour of dialysis, thus decreasing the equilibrium time, will both enhance peritoneal clearance.

The most common complication of peritoneal dialysis is peritonitis, usually bacterial in origin, but occasionally occurring even in the absence of demonstrable contamination. The presence of adhesions within the abdomen can lead to inability to recover all fluid instilled and the gradual development of overhydration; however, the most common cause of positive fluid balance is extraperitoneal catheter placement. Perforation of hollow abdominal viscera, usually large bowel, is heralded by the appearance of massive diarrhea following instillation of fluid, with a high glucose concentration in the diarrhea fluid. Prompt removal of the catheter and careful observation of the patient are indicated, but it is comforting to realize that less than 50 percent of these patients will require exploration. Other complications include hyperchloremia, hypokalemia, hypernatremia, hypoprotenemia, lactic acidosis, metabolic alkalosis, and hypoglycemia. These complications can be avoided by careful adherence to the principles of proper dialysis management. During peritoneal dialysis, pulmonary function is probably reduced slightly, but this may be significant in the borderline patient. Careful pulmonary therapy should be continued during the time of peritoneal dialysis. Bleeding is an infrequent complication of this procedure, but is the hazard most likely to require surgical intervention. Peritoneal catheter replacement prostheses are available to maintain a fistula tract through the abdominal wall between dialyses if more than one series seems indicated.

11.2. TENCKOFF CATHETER

The relatively frequent occurrence of complications with the stiffer forms of peritoneal catheters has led to the recent development of a Silastic catheter for peritoneal dialysis. The softness and the lack of tissue responsiveness to Silastic has resulted in considerable decrease in the morbidity associated with repeat peritoneal dialysis. The Tenckoff catheter is a Silastic catheter with a Dacron felt cuff that is positioned beneath the skin surface at the exit site of the catheter, and that prevents bacterial migration along the catheter tract. Both acute and chronic models are available, the major difference between the two being the presence of an additional Dacron cuff on the model for chronic hemodialysis. This cuff is situated immediately proximal to the peritoneal entrance site. Unless repeated peritoneal dialysis is contemplated as the primary mode of management for the patient with chronic renal failure, the use of the "acute" model is adequate for several repeated peritoneal dialyses.

The abdomen is prepared as for a standard peritoneal dialysis, and a 4- to 5-cm skin incision is made under local anesthesia about two finger-breadths below the umbilicus, in the midline. A special trocar is available to insert this soft catheter, but the catheter can be inserted under direct vision without using the trocar. The dissection is carried down in the midline to the linea alba, where another small vertical stab wound is made in the fascia. Local anesthesia should be infiltrated to the level of the peritoneum. Because of the softness of the catheter, it is essential that the abdomen be filled with a prewarmed dialysate solution, introduced via a large bore needle through the subumbilical incision. Either the trocar or a scalpel blade, held perpendicular to the abdominal wall, is used to perforate the peritoneum, and the patient is requested to tighten his abdominal musculature while the perforation is performed. The catheter is advanced intraperitoneally either with the aid of the trocar or under direct vision. As with the standard peritoneal catheter, an effort is made to guide the Silastic catheter into the dependent portions of the pelvis, and the patient will often feel some discomfort in the rectal area, indicating that the catheter is in the proper position. Bladder or more anterior discomfort indicates that the catheter should be pulled back and advanced in a more posterior direction. Resistance to the advancement suggests that omental entanglement has occurred, and the catheter again should be withdrawn and readvanced. If the catheter has been inserted under direct vision, a stitch of 3–0 plain catgut should be used to snug up the peritoneal opening about the catheter and to prevent leakage of dialysate fluid.

When the catheter is in the proper position, it is pulled back slightly until pain ceases and the obturator is carefully removed. A 5- to 10-cm subcutaneous tunnel is now outlined so that the Dacron felt will lie immediately beneath the skin surface exit point. The catheter is never brought out of the midline incision itself. A gently arcing course usually allows corrections to be made for the patient's size in relation to catheter length. Local anesthesia is extended subcutaneously from the midline incision to the skin exit site, where a small skin stab wound is made large enough to allow the Silastic to come through easily, but as small as possible to discourage infection. A pliable uterine sound with a bulbous tip or a Kelly hemostatic forceps is inserted through the skin stab wound to transverse the deep fat layer along the projected catheter course and to emerge at the upper edge of the midline abdominal incision. The catheter is then slipped over the bulbous tip of the sound or is grasped by the Kelly clamp and withdrawn into the tunnel. Because the Dacron felt will bind if the tunnel is too small, the tract should be dilated prior to withdrawal of the catheter. The felt cuff should be located immediately beneath the skin exit in the subcutaneous fat tissue. No sutures are used at the exit site. The wounds are dressed and dialysis begins immediately.

To remove the catheter, the area around the skin exit site is cleansed, and local anesthesia is infiltrated. A buttonhole incision is made around the skin and is extended about one cm down over the cuff. This is dissected out with a sinus tract, but once the cuff is freed, the catheter can be removed by simple traction. The incision is sutured, unless there is some evidence of infection at the skin exit. In this case, the abdomen is filled with 500 ml of dialysate containing an appropriate antibiotic before the catheter is removed.

11.3. INSERTION OF SCRIBNER SHUNT

The insertion of a Scribner shunt is generally best performed in the operating room, where lighting and instrumentation are complete. On occasion, however, a patient's disease and life-support systems give a practical advantage to inserting a Scribner shunt for hemodialysis at the bedside. Patients whose renal failure does not appear reversible, regardless of the awkwardness of bringing them to the operating room, should be taken there for either a Scribner shunt or creation of an arteriovenous fistula, because maximum functional dialysis life will be sought from the procedure.

MATERIAL

A sterile cut-down set such as described in Section 2.6. Floor supplies: antiseptic solution, masks, sterile gloves, heparin, saline solution, 18-gauge Teflon shunt tips, shunt connectors, shunt clamps, and Scribner shunt tubing in the universal, reverse, and left and right standard configurations. Although it is true that the larger the tip that is inserted into a vessel, the longer the shunt life, bedside insertion of a Scribner shunt should be reserved for reversible renal failure patients; therefore, it is better to use a shunt tip size that is easily inserted, and to avoid the hazards of forcing a shunt tip too big for the vessel. Eighteen-gauge shunt tips will fit most cephalic veins and radial arteries. A size smaller (19-gauge) should also be on hand.

TECHNIQUE

An assistant is essential, and an excellent bedside light should be available. Either the patient's right or left wrist area is selected, depending on the presence of pulses in the wrist and a suitable vein. In general, the cephalic vein at the wrist is the most suitable vessel, but this may be thrombosed from previous intravenous lines. The presence of a cordlike vein mandates against using this vessel, and another forearm vein should be selected. Deep veins with thick walls are most suitable for a Scribner shunt, and either the cephalic vein should be selected proximal to an area of thrombosis or a large branch of the basilic vein should be sought out in the forearm at a location that will allow bending of the elbow without kinking of the shunt tip when it is inserted full length into the vessel. Gowns, gloves, and masks are worn. The forearm is shaved if necessary and prepared circumferentially from the wrist to the elbow. Under 1% Xylocaine without epinephrine, two incisions are made at the wrist, a horizontal one for the cephalic vein and a vertical one for the radial artery. These are made almost adjacent to each other and approximately 5 cm proximal to the wrist crease. The vein is approached first, for this vessel is the most variable and proper venous insertion must be obtained before an adequately functioning Scribner shunt can be completed.

Employing the basic technique described under venous cutdowns, a 3-cm segment of vein is isolated between two ligatures of 4-0 silk, with only the distal ligature knotted (see Figure 2.10). Because the vein lies at a more superficial level, the universal shunt configuration is best suited for this vessel, whereas the standard shunt is usually used for the artery. Reverse shunts are reserved for use with vessels near the elbow, where the reverse configuration allows the tubing to continue toward the hand rather than in the usual proximal direction. Excess shunt tubing is trimmed off so that when the etched butt end of the Teflon tip is inserted into the Scribner shunt, it does not impinge upon the curved portion of the Silastic tubing. To ease the passage of the tip into the shunt, fill the lumen of the Silastic catheter with heparinized saline solution (5 mg heparin in 500 ml saline solution), and apply a shunt clamp. Take great care not to kink the Teflon tip even slightly, for this will break the smooth inner surface of the tip and induce early clotting. When the shunt tip is in place, a 4-0 silk is tied around the shunt tubing and tip, as illustrated in Figure 11.1. Again, care is taken not to kink the tube with the ligature. While the assistant applies traction in opposite directions on the two silk ligatures around the vein, a venotomy is made, using a no. 11 blade in the manner described for venous cutdowns (see Figure 2.10). The shunt is brought up next to the vein to see how it will eventually lie, and a curved hemostat is used to make a subcutaneous pocket beside the incision, so that the curved portion of the shunt can lie comfortably beneath the skin (see Figure 11.1). The shunt

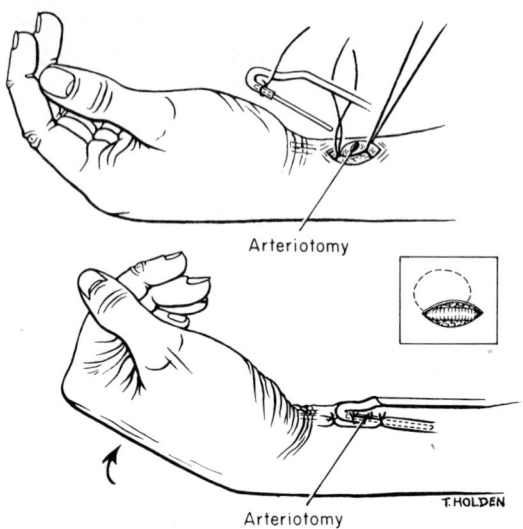

Figure 11.1.

Scribner shunt. To secure the shunt in place in either the artery or the vein, after the shunt tip has been inserted its full length into the vessel, the proximal silk is tied down snugly around the shunt tip and the vessel, and then this ligature itself is tied to the ligature shown clearly in the top half of the illustration, preplaced about the shunt tip and the shunt tubing. Inset: The subcutaneous pocket that must be created prior to insertion of the shunt, to accommodate the curve of the shunt tubing.

is now introduced into the vein by catching the upper lip of the venotomy and advancing the tip. The untied ligature about the vein is tied down around the vein and the inserted Teflon tip. This ligature and the one about the tip and shunt tubing are tied together to secure the shunt into the vessel (see Figure 11.1). Care should be taken not to twist the shunt as it is inserted, and the tubing, when positioned in the pocket, should not produce any leverage on the catheter. The limb of the shunt which contains the tip should lie in a direct line with the vessel used. The shunt tubing is led out a separate, small stab wound. Prior to taking this final step, the vein is irrigated with heparinized saline solution and some estimate made of the venous resistance. High venous pressure will produce a definite sense of resistance when the vein is irrigated, and the patient may complain of pain. Excessively high venous resistance will result in early clotting of the shunt; a new vein or another position on the cephalic vein should be chosen.

The arterial insertion is done in precisely the same manner as for the vein. Should the vessel lumen in either instance prove inadequate to accept the shunt tip, the vessel may be dilated readily with the tip of a fine curved hemostat. When inserting the catheter into the radial artery, the tip is moved slowly and gently. A constant observation for a transmitted pulse to the fluid in the shunt indicates that the tip is free in the lumen of the artery. Failure to see this, or failure to obtain free irrigation of the artery when the catheter is in place, indicate that a fold of intima has been pushed ahead of the shunt tip, and the shunt will not function. The shunt should be removed and reinserted, or a more proximal portion on the artery should be chosen if this cannot be corrected. While tying the arterial line in place, have the assistant hold the arterial shunt in position, for the pulse pressure will otherwise force the shunt out of the vessel. The long ends of the two exposed pieces of shunt tubing are trimmed so that the end of one touches the other, and so that the connector piece can be fitted in without impinging upon the curved portion of either of the two exposed shunts. When inserting the connector piece, care again should be taken not to crimp it in any manner. The shunt clamps are removed, and free flow is allowed. The wounds are closed in layers to facilitate healing over a foreign body. Chromic catgut is used for the subcutaneous tissue, and skin sutures are used as a final layer. A circumferential dry dressing is applied and the shunt clips are attached to the dressing. The nurses should be alerted that no venipunctures, intravenous lines, or blood pressures should be taken in an arm with a functioning Scribner shunt.

Shunts are foreign bodies passing through the skin, and require meticulous nursing care, particularly during dialysis, when separating and reconnecting the two shunt ends. Wound infections with shunts in place can often be successfully treated with antibiotics and need not necessarily result in shunt removal. Shunt clotting is the inevitable fate of all shunts, but early clotting can often be reversed by flushing of the shunt with heparinized saline solution and aspiration. The earlier a clot is discovered, the better the chances for its removal. Nurses should have a regular schedule for listening over the venous end of a shunt for the typical rushing sound that indicates shunt patency. A solution of fibrinolysin flushed into the arterial or venous limb of the shunt can frequently dissolve small clots, but this is a painful procedure, occasionally associated with allergic reactions. Shunt lines that clot repeatedly can occasionally be coaxed along for several additional dialyses by filling both limbs of the shunt with heparin in the concentration of 1 mg/ml and leaving the shunt clamped. No blood is allowed to flow through the shunt, but the heparin instillation into both limbs is repeated every 4 hours. The availability of a shunt connector with a side arm makes this type of heparin instillation much simpler and safer.

12.

DRESSING CARE

12.1. INCISION AND WOUND CARE

The sterilized dressing kit is a very useful unit which may contain as simple an array of instruments as a pair of scissors, blunt forceps, Kelly clamp, and gauze sponges. These instruments will enable the doctor to remove sutures, change dressings, or accomplish the standard care of almost every type of incision without contamination. Although gloves and mask for the physician are superfluous for the removal of skin sutures, *they should be used for every other manipulation of a wound or incision.* These precautions, combined with meticulous aseptic techniques and hand-washing between patients, protect not only the patient but the doctor as well, and prevent one of the classic modes of spread of intrahospital infection: the contaminated hands of the surgeon.

The opened wrapping of the kit may be used as a sterile field, from which dressings and instruments are taken to the patient. Soiled dressings are deposited in a paper bag, then discarded (Figure 12.1).

The dressing of wounds is perhaps the surgeon's most ancient duty; proper dressing technique as an important adjunct to rapid healing has long been recognized, though often underemphasized. Correct handling of bandages be-

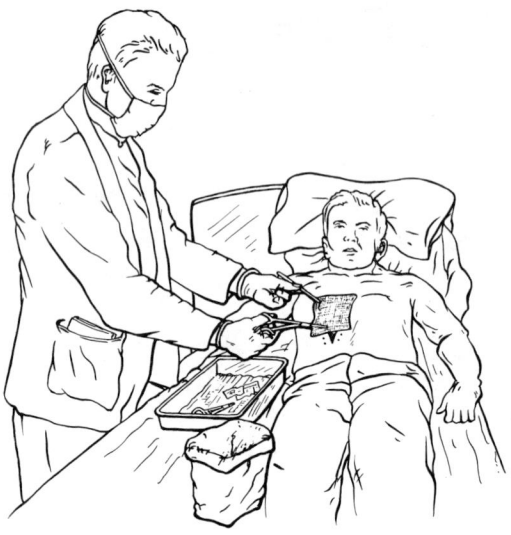

Figure 12.1.

Aseptic technique for dressing an open wound. Wearing mask and gloves, the surgeon removes clean dressings from a sterile tray, using instruments. Soiled dressings are transferred to the bag by the patient's legs and may then be disposed of conveniently.

gins with the understanding that the purposes for which wounds are covered depend upon the type of initial injury.

Wounds with Primary Closure

These include clean, fresh lacerations and the majority of "planned wounds," i.e., surgical incisions. Because the coagulum that forms along the cut edges rapidly seals such wounds, dressings are not required to prevent infection, and may even be omitted in such areas as the perineum, where application is difficult. Dressings do increase the patient's comfort, protect the wound from trauma, and give its edges lateral support during the initial healing phase. They also raise the skin temperature beneath them from about 80–85°F to 98.5°F, and thus produce an inevitable but usually inconsequential amount of maceration along the suture line.

If the patient is enjoying a benign postoperative course, there is nothing to be gained by removing such a dressing until the skin sutures are taken out. This time interval varies. When there is little likelihood of trauma or lateral strain, and when the wound also has subcuticular sutures, as in the head and neck, skin sutures may be removed as early as 3 or 4 days. For standard thoracic and abdominal incisions, the interval is one week. The skin of the extremities, particularly of the palms and soles, is thicker, slower to heal, and subject to more strain. Sutures are commonly left for 10 days to 2 weeks in such areas. Two weeks is also the ordinary time that abdominal retention sutures remain in place.

It is not necessary for the patient to recall the removal of his taped bandage as the most acutely painful moments in his hospital experience. The application of a sponge, soaked in acetone, to the tape will loosen the adhesive to the point of painless removal; this is doubly helpful if the tape traverses hairy areas of the body. When removing tape, one end is pulled toward the incision while the free hand applies countertraction against the skin. When applying tape, avoid excessive tension; this can produce a blistering skin irritation. Tincture of benzoin compound will increase the adherence of tape, particularly near wounds likely to have drainage, but adhesive tape should not be applied to areas previously painted with tincture of iodine.

Regardless of the type to be removed, a suture should be cut close to the skin, to avoid dragging exposed and contaminated suture beneath the skin surface. The long suture end is pulled *toward* the line of incision. The blunt tips and thick metal of most disposable suture-removal scissors make it difficult to insinuate them into position to cut without pulling the suture and causing pain. A simple and effective instrument for this purpose is a no. 11 scalpel blade; it may be painlessly inserted beneath the tightest suture, and it is the instrument of choice for facial incisions and for children, who have an inordinate fear of suture removal.

The three common complications that should lead the surgeon to an immediate examination of the wound are bleeding, fever, and patient complaint.

Bleeding

Bleeding from the incision often manifests itself in the recovery room. The determination of the bleeding site is not always possible, but skin vessels tend to produce a more clearly pulsatile flow. A bulging, discolored incision means major deep hemorrhage and requires exploration. If the bleeding is superficial and not of great magnitude, it can usually be controlled by an additional skin suture. When the incision is over bone (i.e., the extremities or thorax), a pressure dressing will often obviate the need for a stitch. An effective pressure dressing should be firm, and thick, but small. A 2-inch or 4-inch gauze sponge is folded in half repeatedly to form a small flat bundle. This is then pressed inward directly over the bleeding point and against the support of the nearby bone. *While firm pressure is maintained,* the dressing is secured by several strips of pretorn 1/2-inch tape. This type of bandage is exceptionally effective for the control of bleeding after removal of venous and arterial cutdowns.

Fever

The appearance of fever 18 to 36 hours after surgery should lead to a prompt examination of the wound, even if there is a suspected alternate cause. Although hemolytic streptococci are the most common organisms responsible for early infections, and cause a characteristic spreading bright red cellulitis with discrete borders, most incipient wound infections are less obvious and yield the diagnosis only to careful inspection. If incisions are not on occasion to be opened unnecessarily, and infection introduced instead of evacuated, more experienced consultation should be sought whenever doubt exists. A localized area of erythema, seepage of serous or serosanguinous fluid, or unusual tenderness with swelling should lead to immediate removal of the adjacent sutures. The suppuration associated with gram-negative organisms or mixed flora frequently is thin, brownish, and characteristically malodorous. The wound edges are gently separated and the subcutaneous tissue is probed with the tip of a Kelly clamp to find the abscess pocket, estimate its extent, and establish drainage of all its locules. In the treatment of wound infections, the guiding principles are the same as for any localized infection: to secure adequate and dependent drainage. Initial treatment must be aggressive. Although it is usually unnecessary to unroof the entire incision, keyhole openings created by the removal of one or two sutures may not allow free exit for the pus, and undetermined tracts beneath the incision can become abscess pockets themselves. Like water, pus cannot be expected to flow uphill, and dependent drainage from areas deep and inferior to the incision, such as the pelvis, may require a secondary operation.

To maintain patency of the drainage tract, a rubber slip drain or gauze wicking may be loosely fitted into the abscess cavity. Packing the wicking tightly into all crevices of the cavity can block drainage, and should be avoided. These wicks should be changed when they become saturated and are gradually withdrawn as the abscess shrinks. Cultures are taken at the time of initial drainage, but antibiotics are not indicated unless the patient shows signs of a severe systemic involvement.

The appearance of fluid from the incision does not always mean infection. Abrupt serous discharge interrupting an otherwise benign postoperative course may be the evacuation of a subcutaneous seroma, a poorly understood entity occurring with greater frequency in the obese, and usually requiring no treatment unless secondarily infected. A benign swelling suspected of being a seroma should be aspirated rather than opened. Incisions involving lymphatic confluences, such as the axilla or groin, will frequently develop a degree of lymph drainage. Once the diagnosis is established by aspiration, incision and drainage are usually contraindicated, for these measures will favor the formation of an annoying lymph fistula. Pressure dressings are frequently useful.

A more serious problem, often heralded by a gush of fluid from an abdominal incision, is dehiscence. This complication is more common in the elderly, chronically debilitated, and cancer-ridden patient. Typically, the patient has not done particularly well, and has suffered a prolonged ileus with abdominal distension. When the peritoneum separates, the fluid released is frequently copious and of a light pink hue. Whether dehiscence is followed by evisceration depends upon the presence and adequacy of retention sutures, of whatever type. These deep sutures cannot prevent dehiscence, but they can prevent evisceration if placed at proper intervals. Usually the doctor is called to see a patient who "felt something give" while coughing or turning, and then noticed an outpouring of fluid into the dressing. The appearance of small bowel protruding through the incision leaves little doubt as to the diagnosis. A large dressing should be placed over the protruding viscera to protect it, and the patient urged not to cough or strain, as this could extend the prolapse. If strain is uncontrollable, as in a vomiting patient, the doctor or assistant must maintain continuous manual counterpressure while a nasogastric tube is passed. Unless dehydration is severe enough to warrant a delay for intravenous fluids, the patient should be transferred to the operating room.

If dehiscence is suspected, but evisceration is absent, the wound should be gently probed under sterile conditions to search for viscera protruding through the deep fascia. This condition may occur even in the presence of retention sutures, if they are spaced too far apart and allow a knuckle of bowel to herniate between them. The dangers of obstruction or further protrusion require operative repair. Should the retention sutures prevent penetration of the bowel through the fascia, the patient may be safely watched, and usually does not require reoperation. An abdominal binder may offer helpful counterpressure for such an individual.

A persistent draining sinus tract should always arouse suspicion of a retained foreign body, and in a closed surgical incision this is usually a deep suture. Probing the tract with an ordinary sterilized crochet hook is frequently successful in catching and removing the offending material.

Patient Complaint

Complaint from the patient of unusual discomfort should also lead to examination of the incision. Itching is commonly interpreted by patients as the "first sign of healing," but early in the postoperative period it may in fact be the first sign of tape allergy. The strips should be immediately replaced with one of several available hypoallergenic tapes. Tight skin or retention sutures may also cause pain, and the offenders should be cut and removed if feasible. The ends of stiff nylon or wire retention sutures may jab into the skin and cause severe discomfort, if the knots and ends are not protected by a rubber sleeve at the time of insertion.

Open and Contaminated Wounds

Wounds are left open primarily for three reasons: fear of infection (old lacerations, massive contamination during surgery), established infection (incision and drainage procedures), and absence of epithelium (severe soft-tissue trauma, vascular ulcers, burns). Although details of treatment vary, certain general principles apply to all open wounds. They should be considered always as contaminated, and approached with strict aseptic technique (see Figure 12.1). If feasible, treatment of such wounds should follow, rather than precede, treatment of clean wounds, and should not be done immediately prior to entering the operating room.

Open wounds must be handled with gentleness to preserve vulnerable healing tissues, and soft absorbent dressings will avoid unnecessary trauma. When the wound surface is clean but raw, a nonadherent dressing, containing petrolatum or synthetic material such as cellophane or Teflon, is useful directly against the skin. The synthetic materials are made with perforations to allow ooze to escape into the absorbent layers of the bandage. Frequent changing keeps the wound dry and free of maceration. Adhesive ties (Curity), also called Montgomery straps, are made to be tied across such bulky dressings, and eliminate the need for repeated removal of the outer bandage. When first applying this strapping, the plastic liner over the adhesive surface should be repositioned along the inner edge of that surface (Figure 12.2); subsequent dressings will not then become stuck along this line.

Extremities with contaminated wounds should be elevated to prevent swelling and to improve venous and lymphatic drainage. The application of heat will hasten localization of infection, increase the blood flow in the area, and will frequently relieve a good part of the patient's discomfort. Wet heat, in the form of soaks, can also speed the loosening of crusts and debris in such wounds, as well as counteracting a marked indurative response. An equally effective method of debridement, useful for the removal of the adherent crusts over venous stasis ulcers, is the wet-to-dry technique. Fine-mesh gauze, soaked in saline solution, is applied to all crevices of the wound, and is then covered with an absorbent dressing. As the wet gauze dries, it becomes adherent to the crusts beneath, and when removed dry, will mechanically debride the surface. Twice daily dressing changes of this type, combined with removal by forceps of large crusts, will rapidly clean up the surface of a stasis ulcer for healing or graft acceptance.

Wounds left open as a precautionary step may be closed up to 5 days later in the absence of infection, with the expectation of rapid healing; this procedure is called *delayed primary closure.*

12.2. DRAIN CARE

Wound and Incision Drains

Opinions among surgeons about the suitability of rubber vs. rubber with gauze insert vs. cellophane vs. polyethylene as drain materials will differ for as long as there are either opinions or surgeons. However, several guidelines are useful in managing both superficial and deep drains of whatever construction. Although the purpose of a drain is to afford a ready exit for fluids and thus avoid potential abscess formation, a drain is not always effective. Anatomic factors

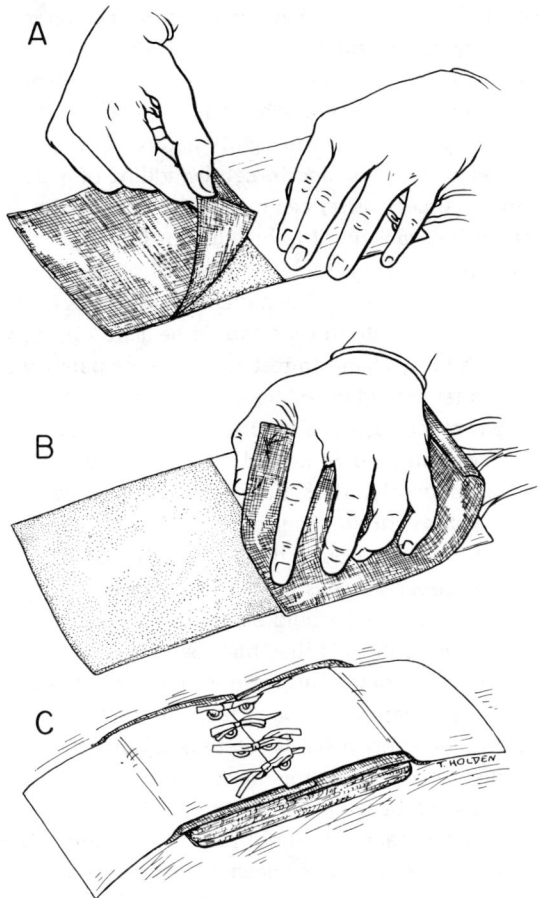

Figure 12.2.

(**A**) The plastic backing against the adhesive portion of the Montgomery straps is peeled back and replaced as illustrated in (**B**). The plastic sheet then will lie over the dressings (**C**) and prevent them from becoming adherent to the adhesive surface of the straps.

may defeat the desired goal; drains led out through abdominal incisions may not adequately channel off dependent areas within the pelvis, or the drain may be separated from the fluid by intervening viscera. When the deep layers of an incision are brought together too tightly about a drain, it may form an effective plug, and forceful wadding of gauze wicking into an abscess cavity can mechanically block all drainage. If clinical signs point to bleeding or infection, the doctor must not be lulled into a false sense of security by the mere presence of a drain. The patient is treated as if he had no drain at all. The drain tract should be gently probed with the tip of a Kelly clamp to test for adequate patency, and small exit sites should be enlarged and kept free of crusts. Gauze wicking ceases to function well as a drain when it becomes saturated with fluid, and therefore needs to be changed frequently. Thus the inner core of gauze in the familiar "cigarette drain" adds body and size to the drain, but the fluid exits around the gauze rather than through it. The rubber sleeve is the actual conduit.

Whenever feasible, drains should be removed in stages over 48 to 72 hours, particularly if they have been in place for an extended period of time. This routine allows the tract to close from the base, before sealing at the skin level.

After first mobilization, a sterile safety pin, pushed through the distal end of the drain at skin level, will prevent retraction of this end beneath the skin.

The maxim that a drain should not be removed until it has stopped draining is valid only for deep or intraperitoneal drains, and even then it is only partially true. Subcutaneous drains will produce a constant serous discharge of varying amounts for as long as they remain in place, and intraperitoneal drains will often do the same. The chance of introducing infection along a drain tract into an otherwise uncontaminated incision is slight, but increases with time. A more sensible approach is to remove a drain when it appears superfluous to keep it, i.e., when the incision is healing cleanly for superficial drains, or when the patient's clinical course and the volume and character of the drainage indicate that intraperitoneal drainage is no longer required.

The use of drains for special purposes, such as a vaginal pack after a hysterectomy or drains for the posterior wound after an abdominoperineal resection, is a highly controversial subject with considerable individual variation. Rules governing their handling are therefore difficult to promulgate with much enthusiasm, except to reaffirm the guidelines above as useful generalities. *It is always prudent to sound out the idiosyncracies of the surgeon before removing any drains from his patients.*

A note put in the chart at the time of surgery, indicating the number, location, and type of drains left, will be useful information for a doctor not present at the operation. Removal of the drains should also be recorded in the progress sheets.

Sump Drains

These double-lumen tubes incorporate the principle of an air vent to allow constant fluid aspiration without entrapment of tissue by the suction. Commercially available in both rubber and plastic, they may also be improvised effectively from a nasogastric tube plus a polyethylene catheter as the vent (Figure 12.3). They are particularly useful in removing copious and irritating fluid from abdominal incisions, as in cases of pancreatic fistulas or duodenal stump leakage, and they are often placed in proper position at the time of surgery if such a complication seems possible. They may also be led down the drain tract of a fistula at a later time. A difference in position of a few millimeters may convert absent sump drainage to adequate drainage, and these catheters should be fixed firmly in position with a stitch or tape. They also require frequent attention for optimal function, including the adjustment of suction strength and the periodic flushing of the air vent with saline solution to maintain patency. Sump drains can erode into large vessels or viscera, particularly in the presence of infection, and they should be used with great caution near major arteries or veins.

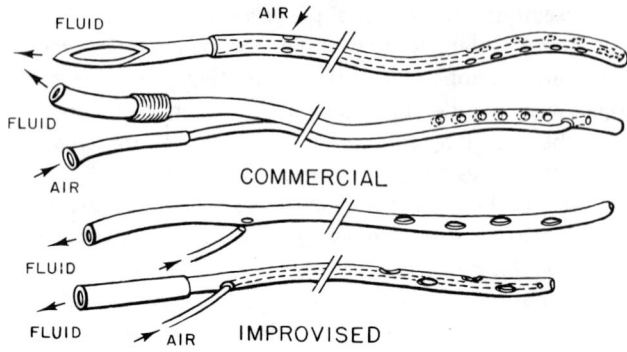

Figure 12.3.

Three different types of sump suction tubes. Two commercial types are illustrated, as well as a unit that can be fashioned from any single-lumen catheter, with a suitable length of polyethylene tubing as the air inlet. The polyethylene tubing is slipped down the lumen of the catheter through a hole made near the flared end of the catheter.

Common Duct Tubes

Because common duct tubes are connected to a drainage unit and are therefore awkward, it is not difficult for the unguarded patient to dislodge this tube while turning in bed or walking. The danger of bile leakage and peritonitis is a real one, and becomes greater the shorter the interval between insertion and dislocation. The patient should be instructed in the purpose of the tube and the need for care, and the tube itself must be securely attached with a stitch and tape (Figure 12.4). A plastic plasma transfer bag (Fenwal) is convenient as the collecting receptacle; it is compact and easily pinned to the gown when the patient is out of bed.

Should the T-tube become dislodged, it is better not to remove it immediately if it appears to be functioning as a drain for the exit of leaking bile. The tube may then be withdrawn in stages, much as a standard drain. If no bile leak is evident at the time of initial dislodgement, the tube may be removed and the patient observed for signs of increasing subdiaphragmatic irritation.

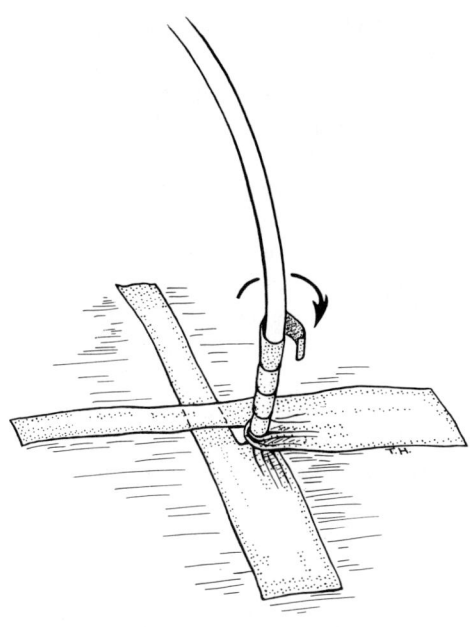

Figure 12.4.

Taping of a T-tube drain or other deep catheter. One-inch tape is split vertically for half its length, and one limb is wrapped about the catheter in a spiral fashion. The other limb and the unsplit portion of the tape are secured to the skin. This process is then repeated with a second piece of tape, laid at right angles to the first.

If the T-tube connects with a drainage tubing that leads to a bottle on the floor, common duct patency may be tested by introducing a Y-shaped adapter between the common duct tube and the drainage tubing, and humping the tube over a suitable stable object, such as a rolled towel pinned to the mattress. The Y-shaped adapter serves as an air break to interrupt the siphon effect of the column of bile leading to the bottle. Humping the tube over the towel increases the hydrostatic pressure necessary to push the bile through the tubing, and thus favors flow through the common duct. Humping the tubing over the bedrail, which is frequently raised and lowered, is neither effective nor safe.

Frequently the tube is clamped for increasing periods of

time, including the full 24 hours before removal. If the patient is comfortable during the periods of clamping, and excessive bile flow does not occur after release of the clamp, these indications are taken as presumptive evidence of unobstructed distal runoff. Finally, a T-tube cholangiogram is obtained on the day of removal. Even if both these tests indicate a freely draining common duct, the T-tube should be allowed to drain for several hours immediately prior to removal, to drain residual dye usually still under some pressure even in a normal duct. A tube plugged by blood clots or gravel is useless, and should be removed rather than flushed out.

Rarely, a common duct tube may refuse to come out. Apply light traction, then clamp the tube with a Kelly clamp at skin level. As the patient ambulates, the tube will frequently work itself loose.

Wound Catheters

Small rubber or polyethelene catheters are frequently incorporated in the treatment of open, dirty soft-tissue wounds, to irrigate antibiotic solutions, saline solution, or one-half strength Dakin's solution into the depths of the injury. Although useful, the dressings over such wounds must be changed frequently to avoid maceration. A sump drain may also effectively be utilized as an irrigating catheter in such situations by instilling the solution into the air vent.

Long, multiperforated polyethylene catheters, attached to disposable spring-powered suction units, such as the Snyder Hemovac, have received increasing usage in the prevention of blood and serum collection beneath extensively dissected skin flaps, as after radical breast surgery. They should be securely stitched and taped to the skin to prevent air leakage or premature dislodgment. Although effective, their small diameter favors plugging by thrombosis; and the multiple openings make flushing the catheter futile. When plugging occurs, the lines should be removed.

Gastrostomy Tubes

These tubes usually are inserted to decompress the stomach after a partial gastrectomy or vagotomy and drainage procedure; as a feeding tube; or as an alternative to a nasogastric tube following abdominal surgery. Regardless of how soon proper gastrointestinal functioning is restored, a gastrostomy tube should not be removed for at least 7 days. This precaution is to prevent intraperitoneal leakage of stomach contents before a tract is established. Gastrostomy tubes should be firmly taped in place (see Figure 12.4), and, because they are frequently moist at the skin level, they should be dressed separately from the main incision and dressed frequently. If a Foley catheter is used as the gastrostomy tube, the balloon may infrequently obstruct the pyloric outflow channel. The tips of gastrostomy tubes can also wander in bizarre directions; inadequate function should lead to a check of the position of the tube by x-ray.

Cecostomy Tubes

These tubes, usually of large size (nos. 30 to 34 French), are inserted for temporary decompression of the large bowel, and are held by purse-string sutures in the cecal wall. They should be securely stitched to the skin, taped in place (see Figure 12.4), and connected by a plastic or rubber catheter to a drainage bag. Irrigations of the cecostomy with normal saline solution can begin within 24 hours of surgery and should be done two or three times a day while turning the patient from side to side. Skin care about the exit site must be meticulous to avoid irritation. The tube usually may be removed 7 to 9 days after a definitive correction of the colonic obstruction, with expectation of rapid sealing. Jejunostomy catheters when used for decompression are handled in a similar manner, but they do not require the frequent irrigations. With jejunostomy feeding tubes, 50 ml hourly portions of glucose and water may be started the day after surgery and be progressively increased thereafter.

12.3. STOMA CARE

Proper care of his intestinal stoma must be learned by the patient prior to discharge from the hospital if long-term success is to be anticipated. This care begins with preoperative education. With encouragement from his doctor and nursing staff, the patient can usually be made to realize that an ileostomy or colostomy is not a pronouncement of life-long social isolation and personal misery. A visit by another patient with a well-functioning stoma or a member of a stoma club will often relieve much of the anxiety. The patient should be made aware of the nature and use of temporary and permanent collecting bags. Those undergoing ileostomy or right transverse colostomy should understand that collection bags will always be necessary, whereas those with an end sigmoid colostomy can reasonably expect to obtain normal or controllable bowel habits.

Disposable bags, to be used once and discarded, are often fitted to an ileostomy or end colostomy stoma before the patient leaves the operating room. These are generally made of clear plastic to allow constant stoma observation, with open or resealable ends, and with an adhesive backing, and/or a karaya-gum ring, and hooks for a belt. This first fitting of a temporary appliance is important, and if the adhesive type of bag is employed, the sticky surface should be carefully applied to the peristomal skin by a gloved hand passed *inside* the collecting bag (Figure 12.5). The appliance opening should be 4 to 6 mm greater than the measured diameter of the stoma itself. When the waste will remain liquid, as in an ileostomy or ileal loop diversion, a drainage tube may be attached to the plastic bag, thus obviating the necessity for frequent bag changes.

To prevent appliance shifting or patient movement from injuring the stoma, it is advisable to hold the bag firmly in place. For temporary bags, resin alcohol or tincture of benzoin on the skin about the stoma binds well with the adhesives. Tincture of benzoin compound is very irritating and should never be used under an appliance. A frame of 2-inch Micropore tape applied to the edges of the adhesive

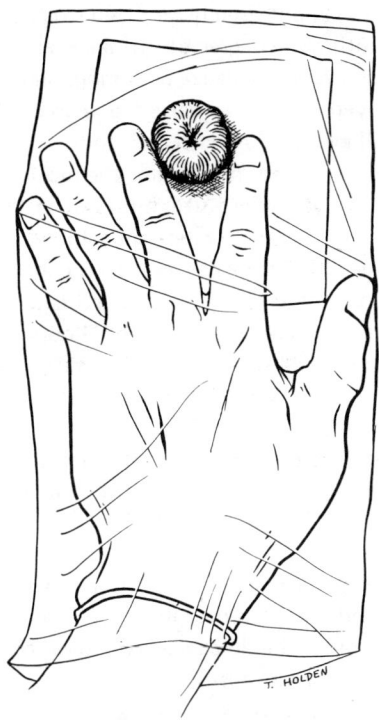

Figure 12.5.

Placement of a temporary collecting bag. Note that the hand is inside the bag and that pressure is applied in close proximity to the stoma itself. Adherence of the adhesive to the skin is most important where it is in immediate proximity to the stoma.

backing adds support with minimal irritation. Elastic belts are available for both disposable and reusable bags. Fitted snugly, they can be of prime importance in preventing appliance shifts, particularly at night. The stronger and more durable rubber cements and silicone adhesives are better suited than resin adhesives for permanent ileostomy bags. A patch test should precede the use of any adhesive, and for some individuals, double-faced adhesive discs will be easier to employ than any liquid or spray cement.

Bulky stomas, such as loop or double-ended colostomies,

with or without a glass rod, cannot usually be fitted except with a special appliance until some degree of shrinkage and healing has occurred. Circumferential gauze wrappings and heavy dressings are employed during this period, and an oversize collecting bag will eventually be needed. In this category, the right transverse colostomy remains the most difficult to manage, not only because of size, but also because of the constant flow of liquid, irritating, malodorous feces. Up to a diameter of 5-1/2 inches, however, commercially available loop colostomy sets with karaya sheets can be adapted to oversize, odor-profb plastic bags. Loop colostomies are not opened for 24 to 48 hours after surgery, unless there is marked distension. This allows the incision to become sealed. The colostomy is opened by a 3-cm transverse incision across the antimesenteric border of the bowel, employing the cautery or scalpel. Full division of the bowel and removal of the glass rod is delayed until the wound is fully healed and the sutures removed.

Reusable bags, usually of natural or synthetic rubber, are made to last for months, and are worn over ileostomies and ileal loop diversions. The rigid or flexible face plate to which these bags are fitted contains a hole, custom fitted to the size of the patient's stoma. The measurements may be taken by the surgeon as soon as the edema of the stoma subsides, ordinarily about the tenth to twelfth postoperative day. Because ileostomy drainage is high in digestive enzyme content, and thus hazardous to normal skin, the hole should be sized so as to leave only a 2 to 3 mm margin at all points around the circumference of the stoma, regardless of its shape. Because of the firmness of even the flexible face plates, possible pressure points on the nearby bony landmarks of the pubis, iliac crest, and costal margin must be considered when planning conformation and diameter. An alternative and perhaps more desirable schedule is to fit the reusable bag one week after surgery, to allow the patient to become familiar with it before discharge. A new face plate may then be ordered at a later time when edema has subsided. Firm adherence of the face plate to the skin is necessary for skin protection and avoidance of odor. Therefore, a doubly adhesive foam disc is usually inserted between the face plate and the skin, or the face plate is covered with ileostomy cement, with or without karaya powder added. The length of time that an ileostomy face plate can be worn will have to be determined individually by the patient. The patient with an ileostomy should be instructed that skin irritations require attention, because neglected lesions will surely become worse. At least two reusable bags and belts should be ordered for each patient, allowing him to wash and dry one while wearing the other. Disposable bags are used longterm, when required, for colostomies.

The natural gum resin, karaya gum, is undoubtedly the most important single item in proper stoma care. It is available as a powder or in discs or sheets of karaya and glycerine. It is the one material that may be safely placed on raw, irritated peristomal skin, then have an appliance cemented over it, and yet allow re-epithelialization. When applied over moist skin, or burned and weeping skin, it forms a tenacious, gummy film that ileal discharge or feces cannot penetrate or quickly wash away. Ileostomy cement will adhere to it. Nonallergenic and rarely sensitizing, it may also be used as a disc or washer around the stoma. These discs on disposable bags are particularly useful around wet colostomy stomas; they eliminate the need for very accurate appliance measurement because they can be made to fit snugly about the mucosa, thus leaving no skin exposed to corrosive wastes. Karaya gum sheets may also be tailored to protect even the difficult loop colostomy, and still allow application of a collecting device. A viscous mixture of karaya powder and glycerine, applied circumferentially about the stoma, can allow a collecting bag to be safely attached for several days when the stoma is located on a fatty fold, near a bony prominence, or is otherwise in a location that would not permit snug application. For ileal bladders, Colly-Seel discs are more resistant than karaya to the dissolving action of urine, and hence are more suitable.

Despite meticulous care and proper appliances, peristomal skin will remain vulnerable. Local hygiene should be emphasized. A bath or shower should be taken each time a bag is removed; even though soap and water do not harm stomas, soap, and particularly hexachlorophene, left on the peristomal skin will interfere with the adhesives and will irritate the skin. It is not essential to remove all old skin cement when changing an appliance. Although the solvent is not irritating, overly generous use of it combined with harsh scrubbing will abrade the skin surface. General cleanliness and removal of the bulk of the old cement is all that is required. Minor skin irritations may be treated by either an antibacterial or antifungal powder or cream, or by aluminum hydroxide, but ointments (including petroleum jelly), will interfere with the adhesives. Such slight lesions will often heal while the appliance is still worn. Fistulas, peristomal abscess, or stomal laceration, on the other hand, require surgical attention, and at least a temporary change in appliance. A stoma that needs finger dilatation to function also needs revision. A malfunctioning or leaking appliance is intolerable; it must be treated with immediate appliance change.

The uniform difficulties of appliance slippage, leakage, and ultimate skin erosion associated with a flush or funnel ileostomy have led to the widespread adoption of the practice of creating mature ileostomy stomas, which protrude for several centimeters. Flush colostomy stomas, however, may be preferred. Ileal loop diversions in general are managed like ileostomies, with certain modifications of the pouch.

Because the first movements from a sigmoid colostomy stoma are usually liquid, the patient with such a stoma should be fitted with a disposable bag in the operating room, even if the stoma is eventually to be controlled by irrigations. Disposable bags are large enough to encompass almost any size stoma, and may be cut to size and fitted over a karaya ring. The first irrigation should be supervised by the surgeon and the next several by trained medical personnel. Most sigmoid colostomy stomas will eventually require only a gauze pad dressing held in place by a belt. Preferably, the bowels should move only at the time of irrigations, every second or third day. This mild degree of constipation should be explained as desirable and not injurious to health. Diet and proper irrigations can usually accomplish the desired results.

The following practical points will assist the patient in colostomy irrigations, if this is the chosen method for obtaining regularity of bowel movements. Because each colostomy will develop a pattern that is individual, it is best not to approach the problem with any conceptual rigidity. Natural evacuation can often be satisfactory, particularly with dietary regulation. Also, colostomy suppositories on occasion can be effective in producing a regular bowel movement. The patient should be made to understand that temporary omission of a routine will not be harmful.

If irrigation is the chosen method, an irrigating bag with a long tube, and a cone-shaped tip to introduce the water into the colostomy, is the more preferable appliance. If a catheter is used, side hole drainage as well as end hole drainage should be cut into the final inch of the catheter, and the proper catheter size determined by the physician. A sheath is used to carry the irrigation returns into a toilet. This is a plastic bag that allows introduction of the catheter or cone into the colostomy through a valve at the top of the bag, but returns the drainage into the toilet. Irrigations may be more successful if they follow a large meal or hot or cold drink. The patient is seated on the toilet with the sheath in place or on a chair next to the toilet. One quart of room-temperature or lukewarm water is placed in the irrigating bag, which is hung so that the bottom of the bag is at shoulder level when the patient is seated. The cone or catheter is lubricated with a water-soluble lubricant, and the tubing is unclamped to start the water running before insertion. The cone is inserted to, but not beyond, its widest point, or as far as it will go with comfort, or the catheter is inserted about 2 inches in the direction indicated by the physician's directions. A catheter is never forced, but passage may be facilitated by twirling the tube between thumb and forefinger. Water is allowed to run slowly, for about 3 to 5 minutes. If stool appears during the time the water is running in, the tube should be clamped and the cone or catheter removed. Some individuals require up to a quart and a half for adequate irrigation, but this is usually a maximum. Cramps or nausea during fluid introduction usually indicate too rapid a flow, while cramps following instillation often precede the beginning of bowel evacuation. Full emptying requires about 45 minutes, but as soon as the major portion has been evacuated, the bottom of the irrigating sleeve may be clamped while the patient bathes or moves about as desired. Bending forward or massaging the abdomen may increase the completeness of the evacuation.

Whatever the type of appliance used, the patient's first attempts to apply it himself are crucial, not only for the safety of the peristomal skin, but also for the development of his ultimate attitude toward this new arrangement. Proper fitting must be demonstrated by the surgeon, and the first efforts should be supervised by him or by experienced assistants. An extra day in the hospital, learning the correct usage of all the components of his new appliance, is time well spent.

The inevitable odor of fecal wastes and appliances depends in part upon the food eaten, and its bacterial fermentation. The patient will control his diet accordingly, but the use of bismuth subcarbonate, or bismuth subgallate, 0.6 gm 3 times a day with meals, can have a striking effect in reducing odor. Chlorophyll and charcoal tablets are of little help. Commercial products, placed in the pouch, are also useful (sodium benzoate, 20 drops, or 0.6 gm aspirin, crushed and dissolved), and frequent, meticulous cleansing and drying of the pouch are important.

It is clear that the bewildering assortment of ostomy appliances and accessories can leave the physician confused about patient education. In addition, the physician often lacks the experience to counsel the patient properly about long-term stomal management techniques, such as for irrigation, diet, odor control, etc. The enterostomal therapist, usually a nurse specifically trained in the management of permanent stomas, has achieved a position of paramount importance in patient and staff education. Most large hospitals have such a trained individual on the nursing staff, and the earlier a consultation is made to this therapist, the more trouble free will be the patient's adaptation to the stoma. The additional role for this specialist of nursing and physician staff education is of equal importance. Except for complicated cases, most patient education can be managed by the floor nursing staff and the patient's doctor. For difficulties encountered once discharged from the hospital, the patient and his doctor can obtain experienced help from local branches of the American Cancer Society and its ostomy association affiliates.

13.

TECHNIQUES OF RESUSCITATION

When the combination of large hospital size and unusual professional interest have coincided, the art and mechanics of emergency resuscitation have approached the rank of a medical subspecialty. An expert team of physicians, equipped with mobile monitoring units, are on constant alert. It is not surprising that the greatest success in the treatment of cardiopulmonary arrest, as well as the most valuable information about the pathophysiology of this complication, have come from these teams. Many hospitals, however, have adopted two critical measures that have facilitated their ability to handle resuscitation: the assignment of a member of the anesthesia department to cover these emergencies and provide respiratory assistance; and the provision of emergency carts on each floor containing equipment reserved for resuscitation, and in the use of which the floor nurses are familiar. Every physician with clinical responsibility should not only be adept in the proper handling of this equipment, but should also be prepared to assume responsibility for resuscitative management.

No aspect of bedside care places greater mental, physical, and emotional strain on the physician than emergency resuscitation, with its clear life-or-death endpoints. Yet it is essential that a single individual be in command of the resuscitative attempt, if the milling personnel that inevitably surround these dramas, anxious to help but often unsure of what to do, are to be utilized effectively. For all practical purposes that individual is the first doctor on the scene, who should be prepared to organize and direct the efforts of an on-the-spot team until resuscitation is successful or abandoned, or until he is relieved by a more senior physician. The following outline, listing the subject order for this chapter, can also serve as a reasonable chronological framework for most resuscitations. (1) Establish the diagnosis of cardiopulmonary arrest. (2) Decide whether resuscitation is warranted. (3) Establish an airway and begin positive pressure ventilation. (4) Begin external cardiac compression. (5) Secure an intravenous catheter for appropriate drugs. Intracardiac injections if required. (6) Electrocardiograph diagnosis followed by appropriate electric shock therapy. (7) Decide whether to convert to internal cardiac massage. (8) Postresuscitation care.

1. ESTABLISH THE DIAGNOSIS OF CARDIOPULMONARY ARREST

The greatest sense of urgency must pervade all aspects of the management of emergency resuscitation. The absence of spontaneous breathing or cardiac action is rapidly appreciable by the stethoscope. A single, sharp midsternal blow, using the fleshy, bottom portion of the closed fist from a height of 8 to 12 inches, produces a small electrical stimulus in a heart that is still reactive. It has been shown capable of terminating a prolonged Stokes-Adams attack or converting rapid ventricular tachycardia to a normal pulse. Therefore, in a witnessed arrest or an arrest occurring in a patient on monitor, such a maneuver is indicated. When the heart has suffered an unknown period of anoxic arrest, the value of this blow has not been established, nor is it a substitute for effective external cardiac compression. It also is not currently recommended for use in children. Effective resuscitation should not be delayed by more than the time required to deliver a single blow.

2. DECIDE WHETHER RESUSCITATION IS WARRANTED

This decision must be based on two variables: the patient's general condition, and his immediate state when first seen.

It is inevitable in any large hospital that the doctor called to direct the resuscitation of a patient will on occasion not know him. The "successful" reviving of a patient with advanced malignancy, irreversible dementia, or other terminal condition represents the misuse of a facility. If this is to be avoided, the basic decision against resuscitation must be made *before the event* by the physician in charge of the case, either verbally or in writing, so that the floor nurses are aware of it. Under the press of an emergency, a doctor cannot reasonably be expected to withhold therapy from a stranger. If such direction is lacking, he should question the nurses about the patient's diagnosis (this is useful information in any resuscitation), and have the responsible physician contacted at once for orders, but he should start resuscitation if it seems feasible.

The most important variable influencing the degree of central nervous system damage produced before resuscitation begins is the state of the patient's oxygenation immediately prior to the arrest. The routine use of oxygen therapy for patients in intensive care units has been credited with preventing brain damage following even prolonged resuscitative efforts. Dilated and fixed pupils in a patient with a suspected period of cardiac arrest exceeding 5 minutes is generally a grave prognostic sign. When the time period approaches 10 minutes, resuscitation is probably not indicated, although rare survivals have been reported in such cases. Age is another important variable; it is well known that the young tolerate cerebral anoxia better than the old, perhaps reflecting the superiority of their basal oxygenation.

3. ESTABLISH AN AIRWAY AND BEGIN POSITIVE PRESSURE VENTILATION

Although bag-valve-mask ventilators such as the Ambu-Ruben bag (Figure 13.1) should be immediately available on all floors and in the emergency ward, resuscitation should not be delayed while such equipment is being gathered.

To clear airway obstruction caused by relaxed glottic structures when the neck is flexed on the chest, the resuscitator, standing beside the victim's head, places a hand behind the neck and raises it, while simultaneously pressing down on the forehead to obtain maximum extension (Figure 13.2B). This position is reinforced by placing a rolled towel or pillow behind the shoulder. Any dental plates are rapidly removed, the patient's nostrils are pinched closed with the hand not holding the neck extended, and a tight seal is made with the mouth of the resuscitator around the victim's mouth as he blows into it. After forceful inspiration, he removes his mouth and allows exhalation to occur passively. The chest is observed to ensure adequate air exchange; in addition, the physician can feel in his own air passages resistance and compliance of the victim's lungs as they expand. The recommended initial ventilatory maneuver is 4 quick full breaths without allowing time for full lung deflation between breaths. Mouth-to-nose ventilation is more effective on occasions when it is impossible to open the vic-

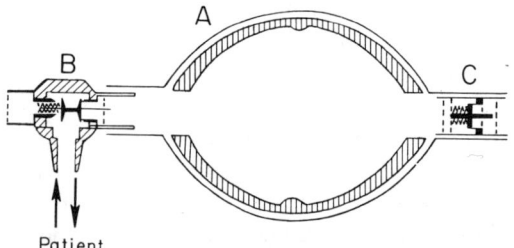

Figure 13.1.

Ambu-Ruben resuscitator. **A**, Reservoir bag with sponge rubber lining; **B**, ruben ventilating valve; **C**, one-way valve to source of gas input.

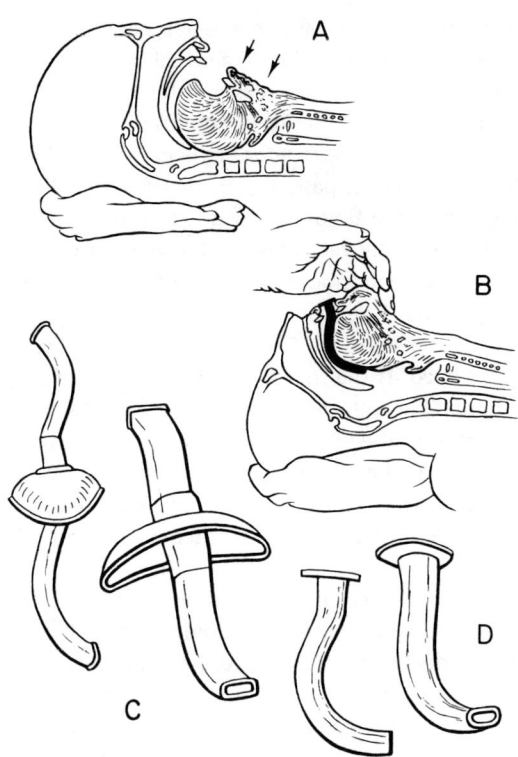

Figure 13.2.

(**A**) The unconscious patient with flexed head and relaxed glottis may suffer airway obstruction from the tongue. (**B**) Elevation of the chin and placement of an oral-pharyngeal airway will clear the passageway. The airway maintains the forward and upward displacement of the base of the tongue. (**C**) A Safar resuscitation tube. The reverse curve of the upper portion allows mouth-to-mouth resuscitation with the resuscitator standing at the head of the bed. (**D**) Standard black rubber oral-pharyngeal airway, adult size.

tim's mouth or when oral injury is encountered. In this technique the jaw is lifted to close the mouth and seal the lips and then the physician seals his mouth around the nose and proceeds as above. It may be necessary to open the victim's mouth or separate his lips to allow air to escape during exhalation because of soft palate obstruction. In children the technique again is the same, although the pliable nature of the infant's neck usually makes exaggerated extension unnecessary. The breathing rate established for adults is about 12 per minute, whereas in infants and small children the proper rate is about 20 per minute.

When an oral airway and resuscitator bag become available, the airway (Figure 13.2B) is passed over the surface of the tongue while grasping the tip of the tongue to prevent reobstruction. Fit the rubber face mask of the ventilator tightly about the nose and mouth with the left hand and squeeze the bag firmly. Adequate ventilation will be reflected by an elevation of the sternum. The resuscitator stands behind the victim's head. If the fourth and fifth fingers of the left hand are curled beneath the mandible, they can be used to sustain extension of the neck and elevation of the mandible. The patient should be hyperventilated at the rate of about 20 times a minute, exhalation occurring passively. Most bag-valve-mask ventilators can be fitted with a catheter to deliver high concentrations of oxygen on inspiration. The neck is kept in the extended position throughout.

Although ventilatory resuscitation should not be delayed to search for the possibly obstructing foreign body, if airway resistance appears to be unusual, the patient should be briefly rolled onto his side and a sweeping motion made with the bent index finger of the hand across the base of the patient's tongue in an effort to clear any airway obstruction. Repeated efforts may be necessary, and a sharp blow between the scapulae may help to dislodge foreign matter. Direct laryngoscopy may also permit removal of the obstruction. An airway of the Safar type (Figure 13.2C) may be used, but despite its aesthetic advantages and its ability to maintain a patent airway, direct mouth-to-mouth or mouth-to-mask ventilation has proved more effective in artificial ventilation.

There is little doubt that ventilation can be improved when delivered via an endotracheal tube in place of a face mask. In addition, if there is evidence of vomiting, face mask ventilation may be totally inadequate and may increase the hazards of aspiration. There is also little doubt that blundering attempts to intubate the trachea not only can cause damage that makes later efforts difficult, but can also deprive the patient of desperately needed oxygenation. If mask ventilation appears sufficient by such criteria as chest movement, auscultation of breath sounds, and clinical response, it is wiser to continue it until more experienced personnel are available. If mask ventilation is inadequate, however, and help is not immediately forthcoming, it is better to proceed at once with intubation rather than persist in a frustrating exercise that is a deadly waste of time.

A source of suction is important, and an assortment of cuffed endotracheal tubes, in size nos. 32, 34, and 36 French, should be available. While the patient is positioned, a nurse can test the balloon of the selected tube for leaks.

The neck is flexed on a folded towel or flat pillow, and the head is extended (Figure 13.3B). This maneuver will bring the axis of the trachea, pharynx, and mouth closer into line than if the head is flat on the bed (Figure 13.3A). The fingers of the right hand open the mouth and spread the lips to prevent trauma by the laryngoscope. Any dental prostheses are removed. The curved laryngoscope is the type generally found in emergency kits; it is held in the left hand, and the blade is introduced slightly to the right of the center of the mouth. It is advanced forward over the center of the tongue somewhat toward the right side until the base of the tongue and the epiglottis are reached. As illustrated (Figure 13.3C) the curved laryngoscope is constructed to allow the tip to pass *between the epiglottis and the base of the tongue, not over the epiglottis.*

After the instrument has been advanced a few millimeters into this position, the larynx is brought into view by a firm, steady elevating pressure, and directed forward and upward at an approximate angle of 45 degrees from the face. The epiglottis is buckled upward and toward the blade by a pull on the glossoepiglottic ligament; exposure of the laryngeal opening should never be attempted by rocking the laryngoscope like a lever on the upper front teeth. If there is difficulty in exposing the vocal cords, have an assistant press in on the neck over the thyroid cartilage. Vomitus or pulmonary secretions should be aspirated under direct vision.

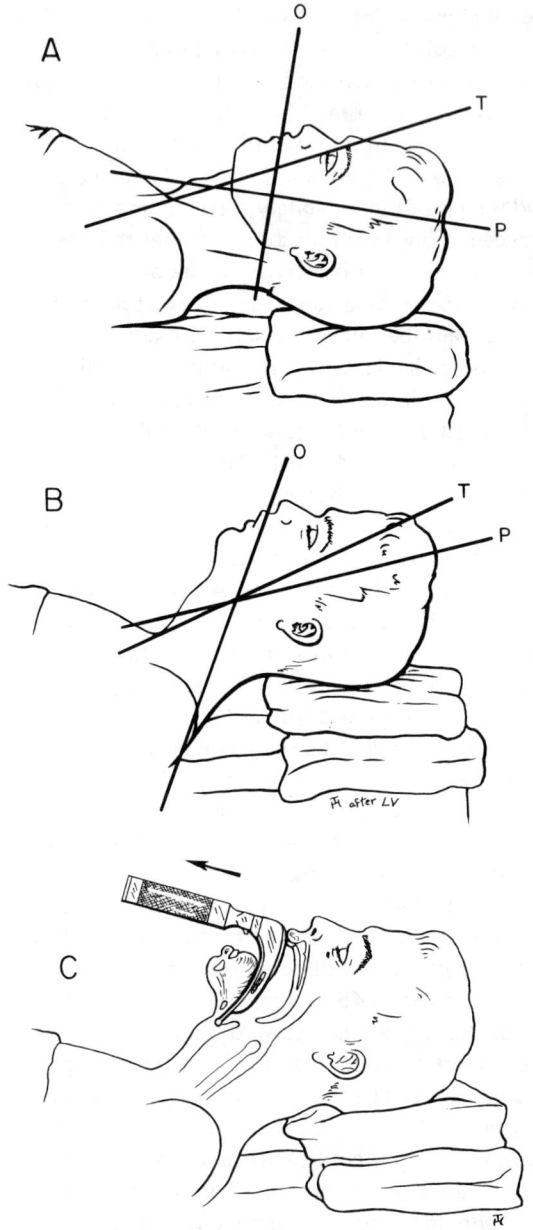

When the blade of the laryngoscope passes the epiglottis and penetrates too deeply into the pharynx, elevation will raise the entire larynx and expose the esophageal rather than the glottic opening.

While the vocal cords are in view, the endotracheal tube, with cuff deflated and its curve facing forward, is passed along the right side of the laryngoscope through the glottic opening and 2 to 3 cm into the trachea in adults, 1 to 1.5 cm in children. Occasionally it will be necessary to rotate the tube through a 90-degree to 180-degree arc before intubation is successful. The tube is returned to the curve-forward position when in the trachea. Exceptionally difficult intubations may be accomplished by the use of a stiff stylet that gives the tube a sharp anterior curve, but such potentially damaging maneuvers require experienced hands.

The Ambu bag is fitted via an adapter to the endotracheal tube, and ventilation is begun at once after inflation of the cuff and brief suctioning for aspirated fluid. Auscultation of both lungs for breath sounds is essential when using an endotracheal tube, for the tip of such a tube can slide into the right mainstem bronchus and cut off air flow to the opposite side. As with the face mask, hyperventilation with high oxygen concentrations at a rate of 20 breaths per minute is ideal. This task may be relegated to a nurse or oxygen therapist once the tube is in place.

4. BEGIN EXTERNAL CARDIAC COMPRESSION

After four or five effective ventilations, check for a carotid pulse. If it is absent, begin external cardiac massage at once. To be effective, a board or firm substance must be placed behind the patient's back; if the emergency cart does not

---

Figure 13.3.

(**A**) The axes of the trachea (**T**), pharynx (**P**), and oral cavities (**O**) are illustrated with the head in the normal supine position. (**B**) Flexing the cervical spine on an extra pillow and extending the head into the "sniffing" position bring the axes into closer alignment. (**C**) The curved laryngoscope passes beneath the epiglottis, and the direction of pull is indicated. This parallels the handle of the instrument, and no rocking motion on the patient's teeth is necessary.

contain such a board, a firm surface may be improvised from a serving tray, or the patient may be placed on the floor. The resuscitator, standing at the victim's side, should be able to lean over the center of the sternum when his hands are in place on the sternum, and to keep his elbows straight. For most hospital beds this will require standing on a low stool. Do not delay massage by waiting for either a board or a stool.

The effectiveness of external cardiac massage is dependent on the fact that the heart is almost in the middle of the chest between the lower sternum and the spine. Rhythmic pressure over the lower half of the sternum will compress the heart against the spine, and produce a pulsatile circulation. To work, pressure sufficient to depress the sternum 1.5 to 2 inches must be applied in an adult, and because filling of the heart will be slow, a rate of no more than once a second is proper.

The heel of one hand is placed over the lower half of the sternum in the midline, and the palm of the other hand rests on the back of the first (Figure 13.4). The fingers do no pushing and need not touch the skin. Do not place the hand over the flexible xyphoid process, which can result in lethal lacerations of the liver, or over the ribs, which can fracture and lacerate the lung. Pressure is exerted with the arms straight, and should be regular, smooth, and uninterrupted. Compression and relaxation are of equal duration, and although the hands are not removed during relaxation, for adequate refilling of the heart the relaxation of the sternum must be complete. The technique for children is similar, except that the heel of only one hand is used for small children and only the tips of the index and middle fingers for infants. The rate for children is about 80 to 100 per minute. Because the ventricles of small children and infants lie higher in the chest, pressure should be applied over the midsternum. Also, the high position of the liver and the pliability of the chest in children increase the danger of liver laceration. Compression should be sufficient to move the sternum about one-fifth of the distance from the front

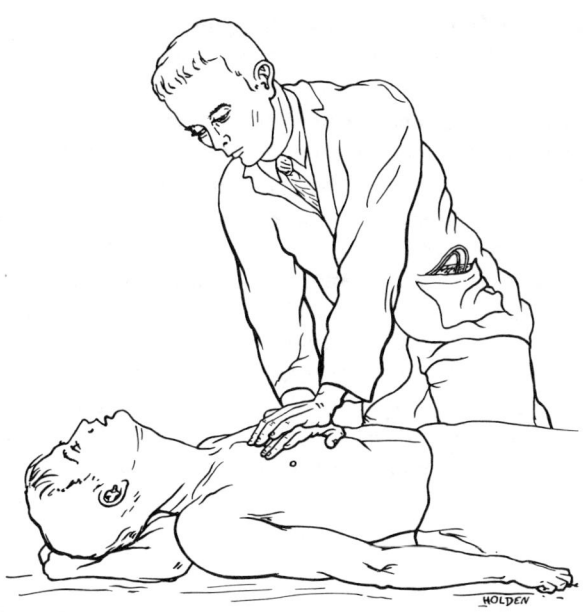

Figure 13.4.

External cardiac compression. Note that the resuscitator leans out over the center of the sternum, to deliver the full weight of his shoulders behind the thrust. The elbows are maintained in an extended position, and pressure is delivered to the palms of the hands, not the fingers.

to the back of the chest, and firm support can be provided by slipping the free hand beneath the child's back. An alternative method for babies is to encircle the chest with the hands and compress the midsternum with both thumbs.

The creation of a femoral pulse is an inaccurate indication of the adequacy of external massage; it has been shown that compression delivered over the umbilicus can produce the sensation of a femoral pulse. Although carotid pulses are more reliable, the state of the pupils provides the best assessment of circulation. Pupils that are not dilated and respond to light indicate effective cerebral blood flow, whereas dilated and fixed pupils connote impending or established brain damage. Dilated but responsive pupils have a less ominous prognosis. Drugs given during the course of resuscitation can alter pupillary reactivity.

Optimum ventilation and circulation are achieved when two resuscitators coordinate their efforts in a regular rhythm, such as a steady chest compression ratio of 60 per minute, without pause for ventilation, while lung inflation is interposed between compressions after each fifth compression. If there is a delay in assembling a two-man resuscitation team, the physician should compress the sternum at a rate of 80 per minute, and after each 15 compressions interpose two quick lung inflations. The faster compression rate works out to 60 per minute when the necessary interruptions are included. External massage is a fatiguing exercise, and if the compression is to be maintained on a smooth and effective basis, the individual doing it must be relieved when he begins to tire. Cardiopulmonary resuscitation should never be interrupted for longer than 5 seconds.

5. SECURE AN INTRAVENOUS CATHETER FOR APPROPRIATE DRUGS. INTRACARDIAC INJECTIONS IF REQUIRED.

This step and the obtaining of an electrocardiogram are usually performed simultaneously. A central venous pressure line at this time is a luxury, although a physician with experience can rapidly place a percutaneous subclavian line (see Section 2.4, Subclavian Vein Catheterization). What is required is a stable route for the administration of drugs, and therefore a venous cutdown in a distal vessel is preferred (see Section 2.6, Venous Cutdowns). The most readily accessible veins of large bore are the saphenous vein at the ankle and the cephalic vein at the wrist. Time should not be wasted searching for peripheral veins, for these will be collapsed during a period of cardiac arrest.

Although individual preferences exist, there is general agreement that certain drugs are useful in the management of cardiopulmonary resuscitation.

Epinephrine

Epinephrine's action in restoring electrical activity in asystole and enhancing defibrillation in ventricular fibrillation is well documented. The drug can increase myocardial contractility, elevate perfusion pressure, lower defibrillation threshold, and, on occasion, restore contractility of the heart in electromechanical dissociation. A dose of 0.5 ml of a 1:1,000 solution diluted to 10 ml, or 5 ml of a 1:10,000 solution is given every 5 minutes intravenously during resuscitation. The repetition is necessary because this dose has a duration of action of only 3 to 5 minutes.

Calcium Chloride

This drug is useful in profound cardiovascular collapse induced by electromechanical dissociation. Its action increases contractility of the myocardium, enhances ventricular excitability, and prolongs systole. In fully digitalized patients, however, rapid intravenous injection of calcium chloride can suppress sinus electrical excitation and produce sudden death. The drug may also be useful in restoring electrical rhythm in patients with asystole, or in enhancing defibrillation.

Dosage of the drug varies and is difficult to codify. The usual recommended dose of calcium chloride is 2.5 to 5 ml of a 10% solution (3.4–6.8 mEq of calcium). Calcium gluconate provides less ionized calcium per unit volume and should be given as 10 ml of a 10% solution (4.8 mEq). The amount should be given intravenously at intervals of about 10 minutes. However, repeated doses may elevate the blood levels dangerously. Also, the drug should not be given simultaneously with sodium bicarbonate, for this mixture results in formation of a precipitate of calcium carbonate.

Sodium Bicarbonate

Immediately following cessation of peripheral blood flow, anaerobic metabolism increases, particularly in the muscles, and this will cause an intense and persistent metabolic acidosis during resuscitation unless countered vigorously with intravenous sodium bicarbonate. A normal blood pH is essential if the heart and blood vessels are to respond properly to the various drugs used during resuscitation. It is administered intravenously in an initial dose of 1 mEq/kg, by either bolus injection or continuous infusion over a 10-minute period. After effective spontaneous circulation is restored, further administration of this drug usually is not indicated and may be harmful. The drug is available either in prefilled syringes, ampules, or bottles of 500 ml solutions of 5% solution. The dosage of 1 mEq/kg should be used regardless of the preparation available.

During attempts to reverse ventricular fibrillation, intravenous sodium bicarbonate is given after the initial attempt at defibrillation. If this is not effective in restoring circulation, a repeat dose of 1 mEq/kg of bicarbonate is given. Subsequent administration of this drug, if possible, should be monitored by arterial blood gases and pH measurements. In order to remove carbon dioxide in the arterial blood, effective ventilation must accompany the administration of this drug. If blood gas and pH determinations are unavailable, one-half of the initial dose may be administered at 10-minute intervals. Although epinephrine or other catecholamines can be given simultaneously in rapid succession with sodium bicarbonate, they should not be added to continuous infusions of bicarbonate, for this may inactivate them. In instances of standstill or persistent ventricular fibrillation, sodium bicarbonate should always be used in conjunction with epinephrine, rather than alone. This combination may convert a cardiac standstill to ventricular fibrillation, which then can be defibrillated. The two drugs together during ventricular fibrillation improve the status of the myocardium and enhance the effectiveness of defibrillation.

Atropine Sulfate

Because this drug reduces vagal tone and enhances atrial ventricular conduction, accelerating the cardiac rate in instances of sinus bradycardia, its primary use in resuscitation is in preventing arrest rather than reversing arrest. It is most frequently employed in cases of profound sinus bradycardia secondary to myocardial infarction, particularly when hypotension is present. In this case, acceleration of the heart rate to 60 to 80 beats per minute may well improve cardiac output and avoid ventricular fibrillation secondary to ectopic electrical activity. When a sinus bradycardia is accompanied by a pulse of less than 60 beats a minute or systolic blood pressure of less than 90, the drug is administered in a dose of 0.5 mg intravenously as a bolus and is repeated at 5-minute intervals until a satisfactory pulse rate is achieved. However, the total dose should not exceed 2 mg except in cases of third-degree atrial ventricular block. Larger doses may be indicated in this condition.

Lidocaine

The antidysrhythmic effect of lidocaine is by means of its action in increasing the electrical stimulation threshold of the ventricle during diastole. It also raises the fibrillation threshold and is particularly effective in depressing irritability when successful defibrillation is followed by repeated return to ventricular fibrillation. It is also effective in controlling multifocal premature ventricular beats and ventricular tachycardia. An initial dose of 50 to 100 mg given as a bolus may be followed by continuous infusion of 1 to 3 mg per minute, usually not exceeding 4 mg per minute. It is not indicated in cardiac standstill.

Isoproterenol

Isoproterenol (Isuprel) hydrochloride is the drug of choice for immediate treatment of patients with profound bradycardia secondary to complete heart block, or with profound sinus bradycardia refractory to atropine. It should be infused in amounts of 2 to 20 μg per minute (1–10 ml of a solution of 1 mg in 500 ml of 5% dextrose and water) with rate administration varied to increase heart rate to approximately 60 beats per minute.

All of the drugs mentioned above can be delivered with effectiveness via a stable intravenous route, and this should be the preferred avenue of delivery. However, in the absence of an intravenous line, intracardiac injections of epinephrine may be given. A spinal 20- or 22-gauge needle, connected with the drug-filled syringe, is inserted at right angles to the chest wall in the fourth or fifth left intercostal space approximately 1.5 inches to the left of the sternal border. Free aspiration of blood indicates that the tip is within the ventricular lumen, and the contents of the syringe are delivered as a bolus. The needle is then withdrawn and external massage is begun again immediately.

It is not surprising that in the hectic activity of emergency cardiopulmonary resuscitation the sequence of drug administration—or whether drug is given at all—can become difficult to recall. To avoid both overdosage with these potent agents, or failure to give an indicated medication, an important logistic step early in the resuscitation procedure is to assign an individual, usually a floor nurse, to the task of gathering together the various medications, and maintaining a running log of medications given, their concentrations, and the time of administration.

6. ELECTROCARDIOGRAPHIC DIAGNOSIS FOLLOWED BY APPROPRIATE ELECTRIC SHOCK THERAPY

Electrocardiographic monitoring should be established early during resuscitation efforts. Standard limb leads may be placed by a nurse during the commencement of the procedure, with lead II being most suitable for diagnosis. One of four common patterns will usually present itself: ventricular tachycardia, ventricular fibrillation, cardiac standstill, or the presence of some other sort of coordinated electrical complexes without clinical evidence of cardiac output. A more unusual finding is the profound bradycardia associated with an Adams-Stokes attack, with complete atrioventricular dissociation. The most desirable type of unit for the emergency situation is the monitor-defibrillator with combination electrocardiogram electrode-defibrillator paddles. Application of these paddles to the chest may be followed by immediate determination of the cardiac rhythm. As indicated in the previous sections, for electric shock therapy to be most successful, it must coincide with optimal myocardial oxygenation and with periods of peak drug effectiveness. During defibrillation, the need for external cardiac support should remain uppermost in the mind of the resuscitator, and the procedure of defibrillation should interrupt external massage only briefly.

Ventricular Tachycardia or Ventricular Fibrillation

The simultaneous depolarization of all muscle fascicles of the heart following defibrillation may be followed by a spontaneous beat if the myocardium is oxygenated and not acidotic. Direct-current defibrillating devices are now generally accepted as superior to those using alternating current. These defibrillating shocks should be delivered as soon as a diagnosis of ventricular fibrillation is known. Countershocks may also be useful on an emergency basis in the presence of ventricular tachycardia without a peripheral pulse. With ventricular asystole, defibrillation has not been demonstrated to be useful, although it is sometimes employed when the electrocardiographic distinction between fine ventricular fibrillation or true standstill is difficult. Proper use of both external and internal electrode paddles will be outlined. If a combination electrocardiogram-defibrillator is not available, temporarily disconnect the cable between the patient and the electrocardiographic monitor during shock therapy to prevent damage to the machine. Although the handles of the electrodes are insulated, the wearing of rubber gloves is a wise precaution, and no part of the operator or of others should be in contact with the patient either directly or indirectly via metal conductors such as a bed frame, during defibrillation. Fluids spilled on the floor around the bed should be wiped up immediately.

External electrodes are smeared with conductive paste and are placed in the standard position: one electrode immediately to the right of the upper sternum below the clavicle, and the other to the left of the cardiac apex or left nipple. Saline solution-soaked 4 × 4 gauze sponges may also be used to conduct the electrical impulse if used immediately, and they have the advantage of preventing hand slippage once external cardiac resuscitation is resumed. Because a single countershock does not produce serious damage to the myocardium, there is no reason to withhold it in the unconscious, pulseless patient prior to electrocardiographic monitoring. It should be emphasized, however, that such defibrillation should not delay the prompt application of basic resuscitation in any way. Unmonitored defibrillation is not recommended for children. The optimum amount of energy for the first countershock has not been firmly established. The output delivered into a 50-ohm load should range from 0 to at least 250 watt-seconds, preferably 300 watt-seconds, for a conventional wave form. This range provides adequate energy for most emergency needs. It has been customary to deliver a 400 joule (watt-second) shock in cases of ventricular fibrillation. However, lower settings can be equally effective, and ventricular damage is directly proportional to the electrical energy used. The energy level delivered through a 50-ohm load should be indicated on the front panel of the defibrillator. Due to the charge storage nature of direct current defibrillators, immediately successive countershocks are often useful because the second shock, immediately after charging, may be fuller than the first. Interrupt external massage for no longer than 5 seconds at a time, and resume it while awaiting electrocardiographic assessment of the countershock.

The paddles of internal electrodes are wrapped in saline solution-soaked gauze and applied, one over the anterior surface (right atrium) and the other over the posterior surface (left ventricle) of the exposed heart. Suggested shock for direct current defibrillators is 20 to 60 watt-seconds over 4 to 6 milliseconds. It is occasionally more effective at these lower levels to give two or even three rapidly sequential shocks each time the electrodes are used.

Cardiac Standstill or Ineffective Beat

Inability to obtain an effective spontaneous rhythm through drug therapy should be followed by efforts to pace the heart by means of electric stimuli. Even in the hands of the most experienced physicians, this theoretically plausible approach has proved generally disappointing, although occasionally life-saving. External pacing requires the application of surface electrodes held in place by a chest strap, or subcutaneous needle electrodes. These are connected to an external pacemaker control unit that has both rate and voltage output controls. Battery-powered portable units are also available. Impulse strength is adjusted until an effective output is delivered.

Emergency transthoracic pacing can be attempted with the Elecath catheter transthoracic pacemaker. This unit consists of a special 15-cm 18-gauge needle that is inserted through the fourth or fifth left intercostal space into the left ventricle in the same manner as for an intracardiac injection, or via the substernal route into the right ventricle (see Section 3.3, Pericardial Puncture). The stylet is of bipolar construction and is introduced once the needle is in the lumen of the ventricle, until contact is made with the endocardium. While the stylet is held carefully in place, the needle is removed. The terminals of the stylet are then connected to an external pacemaker and a dry dressing placed about the wires. Impulse strength for such electrodes need not exceed 10 milliamperes in units regulated by milliamperes, or 4 to 5 volts in those regulated by volts.

Emergency Transvenous Intracardiac Pacing

The ability to pass with speed a temporary transvenous intracardiac pacemaker can on occasion prove life-saving. The specific condition most likely to respond to this technique is advanced atrioventricular block with uncontrollable

Adams-Stokes attacks. Although in theory transvenous pacing offers advantages to external or subcutaneous pacing in the resuscitation of victims of cardiac arrest with standstill, in practice this has rarely proved to be the case. Massive cardiac standstill secondary to a cardiac catastrophe too often responds to intracardiac pacing with a regular paced cardiac beat, but without effective cardiac output. This sequence carries a grave prognosis.

Because the transvenous passage of the newer flexible pacing leads requires some skill, it is better to attempt this initially while not under the duress of emergency resuscitation. The passage of either an atrial or a ventricular pacing wire should be done under fluoroscopic control unless the press of emergency resuscitation dictates otherwise. Transthoracic pacing wires can be promptly inserted by the more inexperienced, are usually of equal effectiveness, and are thus indicated. The passage of a right ventricular pacing wire, without fluoroscopic control, can be performed either via a venous cutdown of the basilic or external jugular venous system (see Section 2.6, Venous Cutdowns), or percutaneously using a Rochester-type needle. The latter technique, utilizing a basilic vein branch, will be described here. The subclavian route is also acceptable for percutaneous insertion (see Section 2.4, Subclavian Vein Catheterization), although not always practical during closed-chest massage. If a central venous pressure line has previously been placed in the superior vena cava, the small no. 3 French Elecath pacing wire may be introduced through this line in an extreme emergency.

MATERIAL

Transvenous intracardiac pacing set. Several units, such as those manufactured by Cordis and U.S. Catheter, come with a cannula for the percutaneous passage of the catheter. A 16-gauge Angiocath will allow passage of most percutaneous pacing wires. It is important to use a plastic cannula rather than a needle, however, to avoid the potential hazard of shearing off the catheter if it is inadvertently withdrawn against the tip of the needle. A bipolar pacing wire should always be used if available, and the soft and flexible transvenous lead is preferred. Although somewhat more difficult to pass than the older, semirigid type, the complication of ventricular perforation associated with the stiffer catheters has been eliminated with the more flexible models. Floor supplies: antiseptic solution, sterile gloves and masks, sterile towels or sterile aperture drape. Electrocardiographic monitoring is essential for proper positioning of the pacing tip. Because the danger of electrocution of the patient is real when the pacing wire is attached to the electrocardiograph machine, care should be taken to see that the instrument is correctly grounded and is functioning properly; as a safety precaution, a battery-operated electrocardiographic machine rather than a wall current instrument is advised. The incidence of arrhythmias induced by the catheter as it passes through the tricuspid valve is low, but it is essential to have a defibrillator and lidocaine solution on standby readiness.

TECHNIQUE

Although either arm is suitable, the approach from the right antecubital space is preferable. The arm is prepared widely about the antecubital fossa, and the field is draped with sterile towels. Gloves and mask are worn. A suitable branch of the basilic vein is chosen in the antecubital space after application of a venous tourniquet. The Rochester-type needle is used to enter the vein. When the needle is within the vessel lumen, the plug is removed from the needle hub to check for blood flow. The outer cannula is held firmly by its hub and the needle is pulled back about 3 cm, leaving the proximal end of the cannula unsupported and flexible within the vessel. The cannula and needle are then advanced together until the hub of the cannula is against the skin. The needle is withdrawn completely, and the plug is transferred from the needle to the cannula fitting. The electrical connections at the distal end of the pacemaker wire are attached to the V lead of a direct writer electrocardiograph machine (set to VI), by means of an alligator clip adapter. Electrocardiograph limb leads have previously been attached in the standard manner. The plug in the outer cannula is removed again, and the pacing wire is advanced rapidly, but gently, through the cannula into the right atrium, allowing the soft catheter literally to float in the venous stream. Difficulty passing the axilla may be overcome by manipulating the arm (see Section 2.6, Venous Cutdowns). Once the lead is in the right atrium, a characteristic atrial pattern is recorded on the electrocardiograph (Figure 13.5). With gentle manipulation the electrode may now be advanced through the tricuspid valve, and the platinum tip will come to rest on the endocardial surface of the right ventricle. Once again the electrocardiographic pattern of the right ventricle is readily recognized (Figure 13.5). After some gentle additional manipulation to ascertain that the tip is secure in its position, the cannula is removed from the vein. The lead is stitched to the skin. An alternate method of ascertaining the position of the catheter is to attach the pacing wire to a battery-operated pacemaker, set at approximately 5 milliamperes, and with an impulse rate 10 to 15 beats greater than that of the patient. The electrocardiograph, run on any lead, is observed, and when the write-out indicates pacing of the heart at the ventricular level, the intracardiac tip is in the proper position.

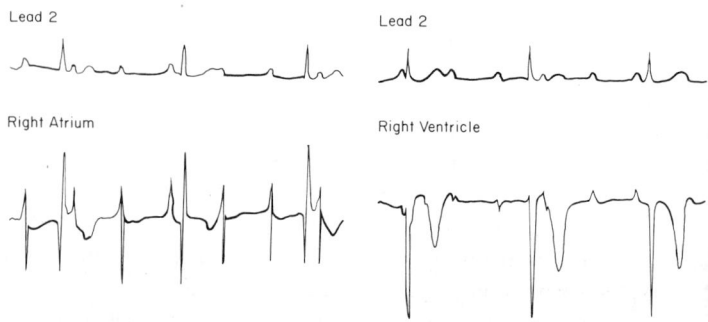

Figure 13.5.

Transverse intracardiac pacing. A typical right atrial and right ventricular pattern as read when the transvenous pacing wire is connected to the V lead of a direct writing electrocardiograph. For comparison, a synchronous electrocardiograph lead 2 is illustrated above both patterns.

Although atrial pacing may be obtained without actual catheter contact with the atrial wall, it requires approximately 2 to 5 milliamperes to induce atrial stimulation, versus the 1 to 2 milliamperes required for right ventricular pacing. It is a less dependable technique than ventricular pacing, particularly when done blindly. Under fluoroscopic control an atrial pacer in the coronary sinus can be very effective, but the catheter position here, as elsewhere in the atrium, is frequently unstable. If ventricular pacing is used to suppress ventricular extra beats, a rate of 90 to 120 beats per minute is usually adequate. Concomitant administration of such drugs as propranolol or procainamide can reduce the rate required to maintain a normal rhythm.

Several transvenous pacemaker units, such as the Cordis, come equipped with a connector into which the bipolar distal end of the transvenous pacer is inserted and locked. This connector is supplied with both positive and negative terminals, which are then attached to the pacemaker. Alligator clips may be used if no special connector is available. Care should be taken that the positive and negative terminals are properly connected. For bipolar units, the negative terminal is connected to the distal terminal. A dry dressing is applied to the entry site and the terminal connectors are covered with a rubber glove for electrical insulation. The pacer is firmly taped to the patient. As added insurance against short circuits, an electric bed should be disconnected from wall current while the temporary pacer is in place.

In addition to the wire's great flexibility, which increases the difficulty of passage, on occasion it will prove hard to seat the tip properly in the right ventricle. Probably the greatest technical shortcoming of this procedure is disengagement of the pacing tip from the endocardium, leading to ineffective ventricular capture and thus ineffective pacing. Although the softness and lightness of this catheter has led to the elimination of cardiac puncture, the interesting complication of knotting of the line has occasionally been reported, although it has rarely led to serious complications. If a knot in the pacing wire prevents its removal, a small cutdown over the arm vein, at the site where the knot is preventing passage, will usually suffice to relieve the obstruction.

7. DECIDE WHETHER TO CONVERT TO INTERNAL CARDIAC MASSAGE

Cardiac output obtained by internal cardiac massage is clearly superior to that of the external cardiac massage. In addition, certain anatomic conditions may preclude effective external massage. The technique is ill chosen for cases of massive thoracic trauma with a flail chest, internal thoracic injuries, pericardial tamponade, chest or spinal deformities, severe emphysema leading to a barrel chest, and tension pneumothorax. In the last instance, the presence of hyperresonance over one lung, plus evidence of an external penetrating injury or the presence of an endotracheal tube delivering positive pressure, should lead the resuscitator to consider tension pneumothorax as a cause for the apparent cardiovascular collapse. In this emergency situation, a large-bore needle may be inserted on the side of the pneumothorax in the second intercostal space 2 inches from the midline. If the diagnosis is confirmed by outrush of air under pressure, the needle should be replaced with a chest tube to underwater-seal drainage as soon as possible (see Section 3.2, Thoracostomy). If it is suspected or proved that one of the above conditions is present, or if closed-chest cardiac compression proves ineffective in rapidly establishing a satisfactory output or spontaneous beat, internal massage is indicated unless the resuscitator believes that a massive myocardial infarct or generalized myocardial disease would cause this effort to fail. A closed respiratory system, preferably obtained via an endotracheal tube and balloon, or at least by a tight-fitting face mask, is essential if the pleural cavity is to be entered.

A careful skin preparation is impossible, but there is usually time to swab the proposed line of incision once with alcohol or tincture of iodine. The chest is opened through the anterior portion of the fourth left intercostal space, and both the fourth and fifth ribs are sectioned at the costochondral junctions. There will be no bleeding. Pleural adhesions are freed, and the pericardium is opened widely, anterior and parallel to the phrenic nerve. In massage of the small adult or child's heart, the one-hand method (see Figure 13.6A) may be adequate. However, with normal adult hearts, the two-hand method (Figure 13.6B) is preferable. A small rib retractor of the Finochietto type will greatly facilitate the insertion of two hands through the incision.

Compression by either method should be so applied as to "milk" the blood from the apex of the heart toward the roots of the great vessels. Prognostic information is frequently available through the feel of the heart itself, i.e., the soft and flabby heart of a massive myocardial infarct or of advanced myocardiopathy. The rate of compression is once a second, and excessive pressure on the myocardium should be avoided. Defibrillation by internal electrodes is described in the preceding section.

When internal massage is no longer indicated, hemostasis is secured, the chest is lavaged with saline solution, and a chest tube is led out through the sixth intercostal space in the midaxillary line (see Section 3.2, Thoracostomy). Several pericostal sutures of nos. 0 or 1 chromic catgut in double strands are used to reapproximate the ribs, and continuous sutures of no. 0 chromic catgut are used on the muscle layers. The skin is closed with silk. The chest tube is connected to underwater-seal drainage. Because of the unsterile conditions at the time of incision, it has been customary to place these patients on antibiotics; it is surprising how rarely they develop wound infections.

8. POSTRESUSCITATION CARE

The frequency with which an individual, successfully resuscitated, suffers another arrest in the immediate postresuscitative period requires that he be under constant and close monitoring, preferably in an intensive care unit. An

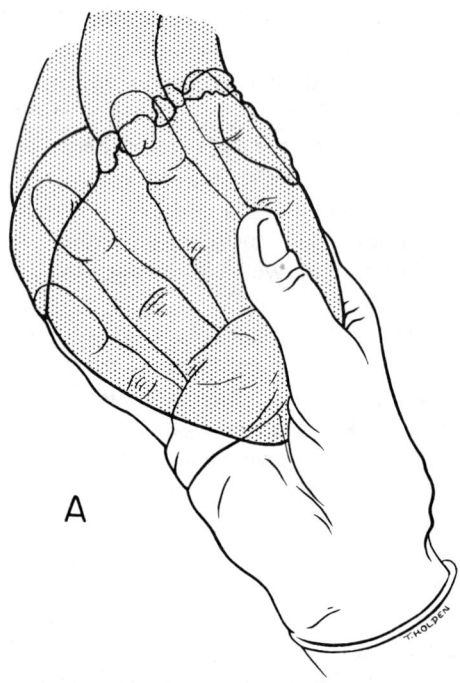

Figure 13.6.

Internal cardiac massage. (**A**) One-hand massage, for children and small adults. (**B**) The usual two-handed massage for normal adult-sized hearts. Blood is massaged upward from the apex of the heart toward the great vessels.

automatic, alarm-triggered cardiac monitor may be attached to the patient to alert the nursing staff of a recurrent arrest. It may be necessary to connect the endotracheal tube to a respirator until the patient's condition has improved and stabilized. A bite block should be inserted between the teeth and tied securely to the endotracheal tube and also around the neck by the same tie. This will prevent the patient from biting down on the tube as he awakens, and because the loop passes around the neck, it will also help to prevent dislodgment of the tube. Tracheostomy tube precautions and care should be afforded the endotracheal tube, and the use of this tube with a mechanical ventilator re-

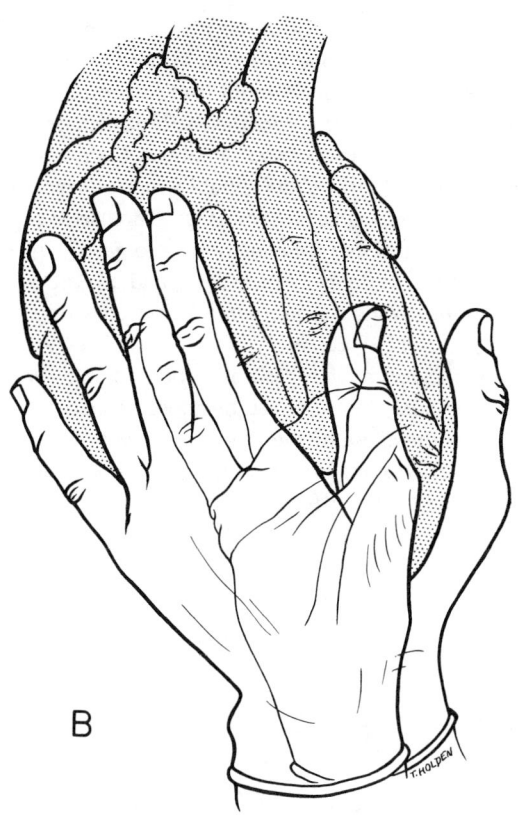

B

quires the constant presence of a nurse. The continued use of vasopressors, cardiotonic agents, and cardiac depressants may be indicated. Blood gas measurements are perhaps the most useful parameters for regulating this therapy.

Most patients should have an inlying Foley catheter in the bladder, and if hypotension is a persistent problem, a central venous catheter will prove helpful. Cerebral anoxia is commonly followed by cerebral edema, and the postresuscitation patient must be watched closely for signs of increasing intracranial pressure. A short course of Decadron (dexamethasone), 16 mg initially and 4 to 6 mg every 4 hours thereafter, may help to avoid this complication, and intravenous urea is indicated for acute exacerbations.

Resuscitation itself is not without hazard for the patient. Evidence suggesting major blood loss should raise suspicion of a lacerated liver or spleen and should lead to prompt four-quadrant abdominal taps. A postresuscitation chest x-ray is indicated for broken ribs and possible pneumothorax or hemothorax. Marrow emboli are a rare but reported complication of external cardiac massage. The use of a bag-valve-mask respirator can frequently lead to gastric dilatation with its attendant danger of vomiting and aspiration. A tympanitic abdomen should be treated by nasogastric intubation.

This list of postresuscitative measures is incomplete, because it will obviously be increased by those needed to diagnose and treat the cause of the arrest. However, it does indicate that a successful resuscitation is not the end, but rather the beginning, of the efforts to save a life.

INDEX

Abdominal paracentesis, 74–79
 diagnostic, 74–77
  with peritoneal dialysis catheter, 76–77
 material for, 74, 78
 sites for, 74–75
 technique for, 75–77, 78–79
 therapeutic, 77–79
Adhesive ties, 217–218, 219
Airway
 establishment of, 238–240
 obstruction of, after tracheostomy, 153–154
 oral-pharyngeal, 239, 240
 Safar-type, 239, 240
Allen test, 47
Allergy, tape, 217
Ambu-Ruben resuscitator, 238
Anesthetics
 infiltration, 4–7
  dosages of, 5
  techniques for, 4–7
  sensitivity to, 4–5
 topical
  dosages of, 5
  in fiberoptic bronchoscopy, 124, 126–127
Ankle joint, aspiration of, 83
Antecubital space
 for infusions, 21
 for venipuncture, 9–10
 for venous cutdown, 38–40
AquaMEPHYTON, 95
Arterial cutdowns, 46–52
 contraindications to, 47
 material for, 47–48
 technique for, 48–52
Arterial punctures, 16–19, 50–52
 material for, 16
 technique for, 16–19
Arteries. *See specific arteries*
Ascites
 as contraindication to liver biopsy, 95–96
 intractable, 78
Aseptic technique, in open wound care, 211, 212
Atrioventricular block, advanced, 253–254
Atropine sulfate, in resuscitation, 248–249

Bag, collecting. *See* Collecting bag
Balloon(s)
 in Miller-Abbott tube, 171
 in Sengstaken-Blakemore tube, 173, 174
 in tracheostomy tube, 148, 149, 151

Balloon(s)—*Continued*
  in urethral catheter, 191
Bandage, adhesive
  allergy to, 217
  application of, 213
  removal of, 213
Barr sex chromatin mass, 104
Basilic vein, cutdown of, 38–40
Benzoin, tincture of, 213
Bile peritonitis, 100
Biopsy. *See also specific types*
  bone marrow, 87–92
  liver, 95–101
  pleural, 101–103
  rectal, 133
  synovial, 81, 83–84
  Vim-Silverman needle, 93–95
    material for, 93
    technique for, 93–95
Bladder distention, decompression of, 195–196
Bleeding
  after fiberoptic bronchoscopy, 126
  from incision, 214
  intrathoracic, in thoracentesis, 61–62
Blood cultures, venipuncture for, 15
Blood pressure monitoring, 46
Bone marrow aspiration, 87–92
  iliac crest, 91–92
  material for, 88–89
  site choice for, 87–88
  sternal, 89–91
  technique for, 89–92
Bowel perforation, in diagnostic paracentesis, 76
Brachial artery
  anatomic dissection of, 17
  puncture of, 16–18
Bradycardia, 249
Breast secretion collection, 105
Breath holding, infant, 13
Bronchi, bronchoscopic visualization of, 119, 120
Bronchoscope
  fiberoptic, 122–123
  introduction of, 117–118
  passage of, 118–119
Bronchoscopy, bedside, 113–128
  fiberoptic, 120–128
    advantages of, 120
    biopsy in, 125–126
    contraindications to, 121–122
    with endotracheal tube, 126–128
    without endotracheal tube, 123–126
    material for, 122–123
    technique for, 123–128
  with rigid bronchoscope, 113–120
    material for, 114–115
    patient position for, 116
    technique for, 115–119
  specimens obtained at, preparation of, 125
Bullet wounds of chest, 68

Calcium chloride, in resuscitation, 247
Calcium gluconate, 247
Cannula, Medicut, 47
  insertion of, 48–49
Carbocain, dosage of, 5
Cardiac massage
  external, 243–246
    for children, 244–245
    two-man, 246
  internal, 258–259
    indications for, 258
    one-hand, 259, 260
    two-hand, 259, 261
Cardiac standstill, external pacing for, 253
Cardiac tamponade, acute, 72
Cardiopulmonary arrest, 236–237
Cathartics, oral, prior to sigmoidoscopy, 128
Catheter(s). *See also specific types*
  arterial, 46
  for colostomy irrigation, 231–232
  feeding, 175
  flow-directed. *See* Swan-Ganz catheter
  Foley, 191, 261
  jejunostomy, 225
  nasal oxygen, 139–140

peritoneal dialysis, 199–201
  for diagnostic peritoneal
    lavage, 76–77
  for pneumothorax, 68
  radial artery, 49
  Rochester type, 21, 24, 25
  silastic, 201
  suction, 141, 142
  Swan-Ganz. *See* Swan-Ganz
    catheter
  Tenckoff, 201–203
  transtracheal cough, 144–147
  urethral, 190
    care of, 194–195
    filiform, 190, 192
    three-way, 190, 194
  wound, 224
Catheterization. *See* Transtracheal cough catheter; Urethral catheterization
Cecostomy tubes, 225
Central venous pressure measurement, 36, 38, 45–46
Cephalic vein cutdown
  on shoulder, 40
  at wrist, 38
Cerebrospinal fluid specimens, 104. *See also* Lumbar puncture
  bloody, 182
Children
  external cardiac massage for, 244–245
  mouth-to-nose ventilation of, 239–240
  urethral catheterization of, 194
Clotting, shunt, 208
Cocaine hydrochloride, dosage of, 5
Collecting bag
  attachment of, 226–227
  disposable, 226
    placement of, 227
  oversize, 228
  reusable, 228–229
Colly-Seel discs, 229
Colonic washings, 107–108
  intubation in, 107
Colostomy
  end sigmoid, 226, 230
  irrigation of, 230–232

loop, 227–228
  right transverse, 226, 228
  and stoma care, 226
Common duct tubes, 222–224
Contrast medium, intraarticular injection of, 81
Cope biopsy needle, 101–102
Cough specimens, 105–106
  postbronchoscopic, 125–126
  from transtracheal catheter, 146
Coughing, productive, stimulation of, 141, 144
Cournand wire introducing kit, 34
Culdocentesis, 79–80
  material for, 79
  technique for, 80
Cutdown. *See also* Arterial cutdowns; Venous cutdowns
  skin preparation for, 2–4
Cutdown set, sterile, 42
Cyclaine, dosages of, 5
Cytology specimens, collection of, 104–109

Decadron, 261
Decompression
  bladder, 195–196
  gastric, 170–171
Dehiscence, 215–216
Dexamethasone, 261
Dialysis, peritoneal. *See*
  Peritoneal dialysis
Drain care, 218–233
Drainage, wound, 213, 218–233
  effectiveness of, 218–220
  removal of, 220–221
  sump, 221–222
Drainage sets, with air break chamber, 195
Dressing care, 211–233
Dressing kit, sterilized, 211
Dressings
  soiled, disposal of, 211, 212
  for wounds with primary closure, 212–213
Drugs
  in intravenous infusions, 20
  in resuscitation, 247–250

265

Dulcolax, 128–129
Duodenum, tube insertion into, direct, 171–172
Dyclone, dosage of, 5
Dyclonine hydrochloride, dosage of, 5

Elbow joint, aspiration of, 82
Electric shock therapy, 250–253
  for cardiac standstill, 253
  for ventricular fibrillation, 251–252
  for ventricular tachycardia, 251–252
Electrocardiographic monitoring
  in pericardial puncture, 72
  in resuscitation, 250
Emboli, from catheters in femoral vein, 37
Empyema, thoracostomy for, 64–68
Endoscopy, 111–136
Endotracheal intubation, 240–243
Endotracheal suction, 140–144
  blood oxygenation during, 143
  material for, 141
  technique for, 141–144
  use of, 140–141
Epinephrine
  addition of, to local anesthetic, 4
  intracardiac injections of, 249–250
  in resuscitation, 247
Esophageal varices, bleeding, treatment of, 172–175
Esophageal washings, 106
Ewalt tube, in fiberoptic gastrectomy, 134

Feeding catheters, 175
Femoral artery puncture, 18–19
  in infants, 19
Femoral vein puncture, 10
Fever, postoperative, 214–216
Fiberoptic bronchoscopy. *See* Bronchoscopy, fiberoptic
Fiberoptic gastroscopy. *See* Gastroscopy, fiberoptic

Fibrillation, ventricular, 247, 248, 249
  shock therapy for, 251–252
Foreign body
  airway obstruction by, 240
  removal of, from bronchi, 119

Gagging, in indirect laryngoscopy, 113
Gastric decompression, 170–171
Gastric washings, 106–107
Gastrointestinal hemorrhage, acute upper, 134
Gastroscopy, fiberoptic, 133–136
  criteria for, 134–135
  material for, 134
  technique for, 134–136
Gastrostomy tubes, 225
Genital tract specimens, female, 108

Handboard
  in direct arterial puncture, 52
  in intravenous infusion, 25, 26
Head mirror, 111–112
Headaches, spinal, 182
Hemodialysis, 199, 204
Hemorrhage
  gastrointestinal, acute upper, 134
  after needle biopsy of liver, 95, 99–100
Hemothorax, thoracostomy for, 64–68
Heparin, in arterial puncture, 16
Hexylcaine hydrochloride, dosages of, 5
Hip joint, aspiration of, 82
Hydrothorax, thoracostomy for, 64–68
Hyperalimentation, 30
Hypotension, postresuscitation, 261

Ileal loop diversions, 230
Ileostomy
  skin irritation and, 228–229
  and stoma care, 226
Iliac crest aspiration and biopsy, 91–92
  needle puncture for, 91, 92
Incision

anesthesia for, 5–7
 care of, 211–218
 skin preparation for, 2–4
Infants
 femoral artery puncture in, 19
 intravenous infusion of, 22
 jugular vein puncture of, 13–15
Infection
 postoperative, 214–216
 after tracheostomy, 154–155
Infiltration anesthetics, techniques for, 4–7
Infusions, intravenous, 19–27
 drugs in, 20
 infant, 22
 material for, 23
 needle in, 20–21
 technique for, 23–27
 veins for, 21–22
Intracath, 21
 in subclavian vein catheterization, 27–31
 suprapubic, for bladder decompression, 195–196
 for therapeutic paracentesis, 79
 for thoracentesis, 56
 as transtracheal cough catheter, 145
 for venous cutdowns, 42
Intracranial pressure, increased, in lumbar puncture, 181
Intradermal injection, 6
Intraflo, 52
Intravenous catheter, in resuscitation, 246
Intubation
 endotracheal, 240–243
 nasogastric. See Nasogastric intubation
Iodine burns, prevention of, 2–3
Irrigation, colostomy, 230–232
Isoproterenol hydrochloride, in resuscitation, 249–250
Isuprel, in resuscitation, 249–250
Itching, postoperative, 217

Jejunostomy catheters, 225
Joint aspiration, 80–84
 material for, 81
 technique for, 81–83
 therapeutic, 81
Jugular vein cutdown, 40–42
Jugular vein puncture, 13–15
 external, 13–14
 internal, 14–15
  for Swan-Ganz catheter, 34–36

Karaya gum, 229
Kelly clamp
 in thoracentesis, 59, 60
 in thoracostomy, 64, 65, 68
Knee joint, aspiration of, 82

Laryngoscope, curved, 241, 242
Laryngoscopy, indirect, 111–113
 material for, 111–112
 phonation in, 112
 technique for, 112–113, 114
Larynx, examination of, 113
Levin tube, 106, 107, 165–166
Lidocaine. See Xylocaine
Liver, needle biopsy of, 95–101
 hemorrhage following, 95, 99–100
 intercostal approach for, 95
 material for, 96–97
 with Menghini needle, 98, 99
 preparation for, 96
 subcostal approach for, 101
 technique for, 97–101
 x-ray studies for, 96
Luken's tube, 115
Lumbar puncture, 177–183
 contraindications to, 177–178
 fetal position for, 178, 179
 headaches following, 182
 material for, 178
 repeat, 182–183
 sites for, 179
 technique for, 178–183
Lymph drainage, 215

Marrow kit, sterilized, 88
Menghini needle, 96–97
Mepivacaine hydrochloride, dosage of, 5
Midsternal blow, sharp, in resuscitation, 236
Miller-Abbott tube, 171
Mirror, head, 111–112

Monitoring, postresuscitation, 259–261
Montgomery straps, 217–218, 219
Mucosal cytology
  buccal, 104
  oral, 105
  vaginal, 104

Nasal oxygen catheters, 139–140
  proper length of, 139, 140
Nasal pack
  anterior, 160, 161
  posterior
    construction of, 160
    insertion of, 161–163
Nasal packing, 159–163
  material for, 159–160
  technique for, 160–163
Nasogastric intubation, 165–175
  intranasal course for, 167
  with long tubes, 170–172
  material for, 165–166
  positioning of, 167–168
  pulmonary function and, 169
  with Sengstaken-Blakemore tube, 172–175
  technique for, 166–175
    water in, 166–167
  of unconscious patient, 168
Needle(s)
  Angiocanth, 34–35, 50–51
  Butterfly, 20, 24, 25
  Cope biopsy, 101–102
  in intravenous infusion, 20–21
  marrow aspiration, 88
  Menghini, 96–97
  Parker-Pearson synovial biopsy, 83–84
  Rochester type, 34–35, 47, 50–51
  Vim-Silverman, 93, 94
  Westerman-Jensen biopsy, 88, 89, 91
Needle drainage of bladder, 196
Needle puncture
  of artery, direct, 50–52
  skin preparation for, 2
Nosebleeds, 159
  anterior, 159, 160
  causes of, 159
  location of, 160–161
  posterior, 159, 161–163
  treatment of, 160–163
Novocain, 4
  dosage of, 5

Odor control, in stoma care, 232
Osteomyelitis, following marrow biopsy, 92

Pacing
  external, 251–252
    for cardiac standstill, 253
  internal, 252
  transvenous intracardiac, emergency, 253–258
    electrocardiographic readings in, 256
    material for, 254–255
    technique for, 255–258
Pacing wires, passage of, 254
Papanicolaou fixative, 104–106, 108
Paracentesis, abdominal. *See* Abdominal paracentesis
Paraphimosis
  reduction of, 192–193
  secondary to catheterization, 189
Parasympathomimetic stimulation, 186–187
Parotitis, "surgical," 169–170
Patient complaint, postoperative, 217
Patient education, by physician, 1–2
Pericardial puncture, 72–74
  electrocardiography during, 72
  material for, 72–73
  technique for, 73–74
Pericardiotomy, indications for, 74
Peritoneal dialysis, 199–201
  complications of, 201
  material for, 199
  technique for, 199–201
  with Tenckoff catheter, 201–203
Peritoneal lavage, diagnostic, 76–77
Peritonitis, after peritoneal dialysis, 201

Pharyngeal suctioning, 144
Phlebitis
  avoidance of, 20, 27, 40
  in intravenous infusion, 21
  in venous cutdowns, 37
Phonation
  in indirect laryngoscopy, 113
  in suction catheter insertion, 143
Physician, explanation of procedures by, 1–2
Pleur-evac units, 67, 69
Pleural biopsy, 101–103
  diagnostic value of, 101
  material for, 101–102
  technique for, 102–103
Pleural contamination, in thoracentesis, 62
Pleural shock, 63
Pneumothorax
  after emergency tracheostomy, 153
  in thoracentesis, 61
  thoracostomy for, 68–71
Pontocaine hydrochloride, dosage of, 5
Postresuscitation care, 259–262
Pregnancy, ectopic, diagnosis of, 79
Procaine hydrochloride, 4, 5
Proctosigmoidoscopy, 128–133
  diagnostic value of, 128
  material for, 129
  oral cathartics prior to, 128
  patient positions for, 129–131
  technique for, 129–133
Protein depletion, in thoracentesis, 62
Prothrombin time, quick, 95
Pulmonary capillary wedge pressure measurement, 31, 33
Pulmonary function, and nasogastric intubation, 169
Pulse
  brachial, 17
  femoral, and external massage, 245
  location of, 17, 18
Punctures. *See specific types*

Pupils, in assessment of circulation, 245–246

Radial artery puncture, 19, 50–52
Rectum
  anatomy of, 132
  biopsy of, 133
  digital examination of, 131
Respiratory techniques, 139–156
Respiratory tract, specimen collection from, 105–106
Resuscitation, 235–262
  chronological framework for, 236
  complications of, 262
  decision against, 237
  direction of team in, 235–236
  drugs in, 247–250
  log of, 250
  electrocardiographic monitoring of, 250
  endotracheal intubation in, 240–243
  midsternal blow in, 236–237
  monitoring after, 259–261
  techniques for, 238–262

Safar resuscitation tube, 239, 240
Saphenous vein cutdown, 37–38, 39
Scalp veins, for infant infusions, 22
Scribner shunt, 206
  care of, 207–208
  insertion of, 203–208
    arterial, 207
    material for, 204
    technique in, 204–208
    venous, 204–207
Sengstaken-Blakemore tube, 172–175
  complications of, 174–175
  technique for, 173–174
Sensitivity, drug, 4–5
  management of, 5
Sepsis, catheter-induced, 31
Septicemia, in indwelling venous lines, 46

Sex chromatin mass determination, 104
Shock
  pleural, in thoracentesis, 63
  venipuncture in, 10
Shock therapy. *See* Electric shock therapy
Shoulder joint, aspiration of, 82
Shoulder pain, right, after liver biopsy, 100
Shunt, Scribner. *See* Scribner shunt
Sigmoidoscope, 129
Silastic catheter, 201
Sim's position, 129–130
Skin
  peristomal, 229–230
  preparation of, 2–4
    for blood culture venipuncture, 15
Sodium bicarbonate, in resuscitation, 247–248
Speculum, vaginal, 79, 80, 108
Sputum collection, 105–106
Sternum, in bone marrow aspiration, 89–91
Stokes-Adams attack, 236
Stoma
  consultation for, 232–233
  intestinal, care of, 226–233
    bulky, 227–228
  mature ileostomy, 230
  odor control in, 232
Subclavian vein catheterization, 22, 27–31
  cleansing of, 30–31
  for hyperalimentation, 30
  radiologic confirmation of, 29–30
  technique for, 27–29
Suction
  endotracheal. *See* Endotracheal suction
  pharyngeal, 144
  three-bottle, 67, 69
  after tracheostomy, 153–154
Sump drains, 221–222
  as irrigation catheters, 224
Sutures, removal of, 213
Swan-Ganz catheter, 31
  placement of, 32–36
    via antecubital basilic vein cutdown, 32–33
    via internal jugular vein, 34–36
  premature ventricular contractions and, 32
Synovial biopsies
  diagnostic value of, 81
  material for, 83
  technique for, 83–84
Syringe, disposable, 16

T-tube, 222–224
  taping of, 223
Tachycardia, ventricular, 236
  shock therapy for, 251–252
Taped bandage. *See* Bandage, adhesive
Taps, abdominal, diagnostic, 74–77
Tenckoff catheter, 201–203
  insertion of, 202–203
  removal of, 203
Tetracaine hydrochloride, dosage of, 5
Thoracentesis, 55–63
  complications of, 61–63
  diagnostic, 55
  fluid localization prior to, 55
  material for, 56
  patient position for, 56, 57, 58
  prophylactic, 56
  technique for, 56–61
  therapeutic, 55–56
Thoracostomy, 63–71
  material for, 63
  puncture sites for, 64, 68
    axillary, 69, 71
  technique for, 64–71
  tube removal following, 71
Tourniquet, venous, application of, 11, 12
Tracheostomy, emergency, 147–152
  airway obstruction after, 153–154
  infection following, 154–155
  material for, 148
  nondesirability of, 147
  postoperative care in, 153–155
  technique for, 148–152
  trauma in, 155
  vertical incision for, 150

Tracheostomy aperture, standard, 151, 152
Tracheostomy tube
 common types of, 149
 in fiberoptic bronchoscopy, 127–128
 removal of, 155–156
 replacement of, 154
Transthoracic pacing wires, 254
Transtracheal cough catheter, 144–147
 material for, 145
 technique for, 145–147
Transvenous pacemaker units, 254, 257
Transvenous pacing wire, passage of, 255–256
Trendelenburg position, 28
Trocar
 Dukes, 78
 Nelson, 64, 65
Tubes
 cecostomy, 225
 common duct, 222–224
 Ewalt, in fiberoptic gastrectomy, 134
 gastrostomy, 225
 intercostal, securing stitch for, 65–66
 Levin, 106, 107, 165–166
 long, gastrointestinal, 170–172
  removal of, 172
 Luken's, 115
 Miller-Abbott, 171
 nasogastric. See Nasogastric intubation
 Sengstaken-Blakemore. See Sengstaken-Blakemore tube
 sump suction, 222
 T-. See T-tube
 thoracostomy, Argyle plastic, 63
 tracheostomy. See Tracheostomy tube

Unconscious patient, intubation of, 168
Underwater seal
 bottle, 66, 69
 portable plastic units for, 67, 69
 three-bottle system for, 67, 69

Urecholine, 186–187
Urethral catheterization, 185–196
 of children, 194
 female, 193–194
 indications for, 185–187
 infection risk after, 185, 193, 194
 lubrication for, 190–192
 male, 188–193
 material for, 187
 technique for, 188–194
Urination, postoperative, 186
Urine specimens, 109

Vacutainer system for venipuncture, 10–11, 13
 components of, 11
 situations inappropriate for, 10
Vaginal smear, 108
Valsalva maneuver
 for chest tube removal, 71
 in venipuncture, 13
Vein(s)
 for infusion, 21–22
 palpation for, 11–12
 rolling of, prevention of, 23–24
Venipuncture, 9–15
 for blood cultures, 15
 materials for, 10–11
 pediatric jugular, 13–15
 selection of vein for, 9–10
 technique for, 11–15
Venotomy, 39
Venous cutdowns, 36–46
 of basilic vein, in antecubital space, 38–40
 of cephalic vein
  at shoulder, 40
  at wrist, 38
 emergency, 36, 37–38
 indications for, 36
 of jugular vein, external, 40–42
 material for, 42
 of saphenous vein at ankle, 37–38, 39
 technique for, 42–46
Ventilation, mouth-to-nose, 238–239
Ventilators, bag-valve-mask, 238

Vim-Silverman needle, 93, 94
  Franklin modification of, 94
Visceral injuries, in thoracentesis, 62
Vitamin K_1, 95

Westerman-Jensen biopsy needle, 88, 89, 91
Wound catheters, 224
Wounds
  care of, 211–218
  open and contaminated, 217–218
  with primary closure, 212–217
    complications of, 213–217
    treatment of, 212–213
Wrist joint, aspiration of, 82–83

X-ray
  postresuscitation, 262
  after subclavian vein catheterization, 29–30
Xylocaine, 4
  dosage of, 5
  in resuscitation, 249